Praise for *Free to Conceive*

An inspirational, uplifting, heartfelt, must read for anyone facing the challenges of infertility. It is like having a personal motivational coach by your side.

Jaylaine Ghoubrial, MD
Obstetrician-Gynecologist

There are so many words to express my excitement for the parents this book Dawn wrote will touch. Having experienced pregnancy loss and pregnancy with birth makes this book even more touching, as well as informative on an intellectual, and, more importantly, heart opening and personal level. A beautiful support for parents in any part of their pregnancy journey.

Mandy Morris
Bestselling Author of *8 Secrets to Powerful Manifesting*

I've watched helplessly as many of my friends struggled with infertility. If only I had this book to give them! It is a total game-changer. Bless you Dawn on behalf of all the parents-in-waiting whose journey will have a much brighter ending because of you.

Debra Poneman
Founder and President of Yes to Success, Inc.

Dawn's heart-wrenching personal fertility journey and the wisdom and vision she developed as a result will inspire and guide you on your journey to motherhood. This book is a gift for anyone trying to conceive!

Kelly Noonan Gores
Writer, director, producer of the *HEAL* Documentary

Free to Conceive

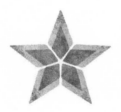

How to Reclaim Your Fertility and Restore Your Inner Peace

Dawn Williams, MA

Edited by Laurie Knight
Cover design by Kristina Edstrom

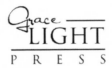

An Imprint for GracePoint Publishing (www.GracePointPublishing.com)

GracePoint Matrix, LLC
624 S. Cascade Ave, Suite 201, Colorado Springs, CO 80903
www.GracePointMatrix.com   Email: Admin@GracePointMatrix.com
SAN # 991-6032

Library of Congress Control Number: 2023937030
ISBN: (Hardback) 978-1-955272-92-6
ISBN: (Paperback) 978-1-955272-81-0
eISBN: 978-1-955272-82-7

Books may be purchased for educational, business, or sales promotional use.
For bulk order requests and price schedule contact:
Orders@GracePointPublishing.com

A special tribute to my devoted husband, Tom, and my precious daughter, Faith, for their constant loving support. The two of you are the ultimate source of inspiration that brought this book into being. I love you immensely.

Table of Contents

A Special Message From My Heart to Yours vii

An Invitation x

Introduction xi

SECTION ONE In the Dark 1

    Chapter One Have You Tried Everything? 3

    Chapter Two Stress 17

SECTION TWO The Five-Point SuperStar System 27

    Chapter Three Surrender 29

    Chapter Four Story 45

    Chapter Five State 65

    Chapter Six Self 85

    Chapter Seven Strategy 105

SECTION THREE Guided by the Light 135

    Chapter Eight Mini Miracles 137

    Chapter Nine Support 149

    Chapter Ten Happiness 165

    Chapter Eleven Love and Faith 177

    Chapter Twelve Freedom 191

About the Author 203

Extra Support 205

A Special Message From My Heart to Yours

If you are unwaveringly devoted to doing anything in your power to become a mother, I dedicate this book to you, my precious soul sister. Your desire to be a mother is so incredibly strong that sometimes it may even feel hard to breathe when yet another month goes by and you're *STILL* not pregnant. The devastating fear of it possibly *NEVER* happening rears its ugly head way too often.

And, to top it off, nobody really seems to understand how painful and challenging this whole process is.

Well, *I* do.

I *was* you.

I *am* you.

I **see** the disappointment on your face and know the aching in your heart as you toss another negative pregnancy test in the trash wondering if you'll ever experience the indescribable—long anticipated—excitement of a positive one.

I **see** you cringe inside when you are mingling with guests at a social event and the third person you meet asks, "Do you have children?"

I **see** your desperate attempts to research and uncover whatever treatment options or fertility-enhancing advice you may have missed that could improve your chances of conception.

I **see** you put on your "happy face" as you attend your best friend's baby shower in your effort to support and celebrate her while you wonder if this will ever be you.

I **see** you struggle on Mother's Day, one of the toughest days of the year now, because it serves as a blatant reminder of the baby you so desperately desire and don't yet have.

I **see** you gazing out the front window daydreaming about how joyous and heartwarming it will be to play outside in the yard with your child one day.

I **hear** your muffled cries in your pillow at bedtime after your husband declines sex with you at night—one of the few prime fertile days in your cycle that month. The wasted critical opportunity cuts you to the core.

I **feel** your deep-seated anger over the injustice of women who appear to be poor examples of mothers yet seem to bear children so easily time and time again.

I **feel** your loneliness as repeated insensitive comments like, "You just need to relax" or "At least you're having fun trying" affirm that no one *really* understands the depths of your ongoing pain.

I **feel** your extreme sadness and disappointment as you notice the evidence in your underwear of the start of your period because you were sure that *THIS* time around you were experiencing pregnancy symptoms and not premenstrual ones.

I **feel** your grief as you are excluded from sharing your pregnancy experience, delivery specifics, and parenting joys and struggles during girls' night out. This sought-after mommy club that you are not a member of feels pervasive in your life.

I want you to know that I see you.

I hear you.

I understand you.

This book was written for YOU and is my way of holding your hand through this journey, so you don't feel alone. You are supported and guided by someone who truly gets you.

I suffered with infertility for six years. *Suffered* being the operative word here. It is my intent that what you will learn in this book and apply to your life will not only alleviate your suffering but will also set you up in the best possible way to have the very thing you want—your baby.

You see, there is a missing piece to this infertility puzzle, and I have it. When I completed my own puzzle with this elusive piece, everything clicked, and the miracle of motherhood became my reality.

Stick with me mama-to-be because this journey you are on is about to veer down a completely different path. One of ease, peace, certainty, and success.

Now, take my hand and let's do this together. I will see you through this to the other side where your baby is waiting for you.

Much love and blessings my friend,

Dawn

An Invitation

Before you begin reading this book, I lovingly encourage you to set an intention. Intentions prepare the mind to have directed focus for reaching a particular goal. Hold the intention you have set as you read the book. It will keep you in line and aimed toward what you want and what matters to you.

To assist in creating your intention, ask yourself the following:

What do I want to get out of reading this book?

What do I want it to do for me in my life?

Here are a few example intentions to get things percolating for you:

- I intend to be open and willing to learn what can help me overcome infertility.

- I intend to feel better mentally and emotionally as I implement what is suggested.

- I intend to reclaim my fertility and restore my inner peace.

Write your intention in the space below.

Introduction

I am so inspired to write this book for you because it is the book I wish I would have had to help me during my six-year-long infertility struggle.

Sure, there were books on the subject, and I did read some of them, but nothing out there gave me what I needed and was searching for—a way out of the excruciating emotional pain I was feeling and solid information on how to get this baby to happen.

Had I known then what I know now, my whole experience would have been different—better. I would have spared myself years of suffering because I would have had the necessary tools to maximize my chances of conception, regardless of whether I chose to use reproductive science technology assistance.

This book, *Free To Conceive,* is designed to expand your mind about what it means to conceive. Not only will this book equip you to identify and clear the blocks standing in the way between you and your baby so that you are in position to be *free to conceive,* but it will also offer you a completely new perspective of what having an infertility diagnosis can mean for you. It may even change the way you think of the word *conceive.*

This perspective will show you that *you are in charge* of how you want this journey to motherhood to go—that you are *free to conceive* how you want to experience it. You will learn to conceive this very challenging circumstance in your life in a brand-new way, a way that will entice you to become the highest version of yourself, which will serve you well in life. In letting go of the pain you have been enduring, you will be able to have the life of your dreams, be it through conceiving a baby, the adoption process, or some other avenue. *You* are *free to conceive* how motherhood can look for you. Anything that ever comes into being begins with a thought, *a conception*. Being intentional and selective about what you conceive is critical. This book will take you on a conception journey like no other, and I will be your trusted guide the whole way to assist you in closing the gap from where you are now to where you want to be. You are not alone in this.

Honestly, I would have loved for someone to sit me down, lovingly take my hand, and tell me the truth about why I wasn't getting pregnant just like I'm going to do for you. I'll tell you about the factors that conventional medicine tends to downplay or avoid, which were no doubt obstacles to my dream of being a mom coming true. These are factors that are integral for fertility and totally within your control.

Yes, it is certainly vital to determine any underlying physical reasons that may be contributing to difficulty conceiving and address them accordingly with various medical treatments and procedures. These attempts work for some couples but not for others. And when none of the medical approaches work or you are unable to afford them—since most health insurance companies do not cover infertility treatments—the road stops there for you, and you are no closer to your baby.

Conventional medicine doesn't really tap into what may be preventing treatments from being successful in the first place and may even be the root cause of your infertility, which is what I refer to as the *missing piece* to this puzzle.

No worries, because I've got you covered with those missing pieces right here in this book! I have it all laid out for you.

Here's a little of my own story.

I was thirty-seven years old when I sought preliminary testing to determine why I wasn't getting pregnant after trying for six months. At that age, it is recommended to not wait a full year to investigate potential physical reasons as to why conception isn't occurring. Doctors uncovered that my FSH (follicle stimulating hormone) was high. They described it as meaning that my eggs were more mature than they should have been for someone my age, resulting in poor egg vitality and low ovarian reserve, which often indicates that early menopause could be right around the corner; we didn't have time to waste.

My husband's sperm also had issues: very low count, low motility, and abnormally shaped. Given our combined fertility issues, our reproductive science team predicted that we had only a 1 to 2 percent chance of conceiving on our own and recommended that we head straight to in vitro fertilization (IVF). We had never attempted any reproductive science assistance before and given the high cost of it, we decided to try IUI (intrauterine insemination) first, since it was significantly cheaper and less invasive.

We completed a total of three IUIs, all of which failed, but each brought with it the hope of it working *this* time and the devastation when it didn't. This really was just the start of the emotional roller coaster ride.

On to the very involved in vitro fertilization route it was.

Due to my high FSH, I barely met the required criteria to complete this procedure. There must be a minimum of four follicles developed before egg retrieval is pursued.

Whew, I got to the four by the skin of my teeth.

During the egg retrieval, the doctor was only able to retrieve three eggs. I was grateful for the three; I saw it as three chances for fertilization to happen so that the next step of transferring the embryo(s) to my uterus for implantation could occur.

The embryologist said to me, "From what I can see, we have three good viable eggs and three good sperm, so I am hopeful that fertilization will occur."

I was working as an elementary school counselor at the time, and I so vividly remember the call I received from my embryologist that next, fateful day.

She said, "I am so sorry, but we couldn't get any of the eggs to fertilize."

I was in shock.

It felt like a death to me.

I felt this was our *one* big shot, and it was taken from us too?

We didn't even get out of the gate to have a chance to transfer the embryo. If science couldn't get perfectly selected sperm and eggs to fertilize in a controlled environment, how were we ever going to get it to happen naturally? We were deflated.

So many feelings were swirling around inside of me. I felt defeated. I felt angry. I felt inadequate. I felt frustrated. I felt distraught. I felt that maybe God was punishing me for going the science route. I felt like this whole thing was unfair. I felt sorry for myself. I felt out of control because nothing was working—not prayers, not science, and certainly *not me*.

I felt so much loss in that one moment. I felt the loss of this baby that I had already imagined.

I felt the loss of all the experiences I dreamed of having,

like seeing that second line on the pregnancy test and surprising my husband with the news,

hearing the baby's heartbeat from in my womb,

feeling the baby kick,

seeing those coveted ultrasound pictures,

embodying the beauty of the miracle growing inside of me for nine months,

having the truly awesome experience of giving birth,

hearing "It's a boy (or girl)!"

having the unique, unto itself, amazingly indescribable feeling of love as my baby is handed to me to nestle in my arms for the very first time,

smelling her sweet skin, looking into her eyes (that I can already tell resemble her daddy's) with utter amazement of this blessing as we decide on the name she will bear,

and, of course, experiencing all of the many developmental milestones and firsts to occur as life begins with our newly expanded family.

So much loss from one phone call. I literally felt that my heart was breaking, shattering into pieces. I truly knew at that point what the word *heartbreaking* meant.

Thankfully, my story doesn't end there.

It ends with me becoming the mom I always wanted to be.

I will tell you more about that later in the book. The really cool thing is that this can be the end of your story too: you with *your* baby.

The middle of the story is where the magic is. The middle of the story is where the missing piece is that I have referred to. The middle of the story is where I went from feeling like a powerless victim of an unfair disease to a confident, empowered, trusting woman who was certain her day was coming. The transformation that occurred and *how* it occurred is what finally made me a mama.

The middle of the story is what this book is about. You will have, right at your fingertips, the missing piece standing in the way between you and the baby you so desire.

Are you ready to say goodbye to the fear and anxiety? To this unpleasant burden? To the stress and frustration you feel?

Are you ready to say hello to enjoying the journey with peace and ease? To living your life without the heaviness of this struggle and being so consumed by it? Are you ready to experience that freedom?

Are you ready to figure out *your* missing piece?

Let's get started then.

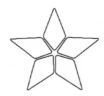

I created a simple tool to help you zero in on your missing piece(s). I call it my Five-Point SuperStar System. The star comprises the five key components that play a critical role in the level of success and happiness we experience in life. It is when all five of these components are synchronized that we feel in flow, and life seems easy. One or more points of this star are likely out of sync for you right now and identifying which ones they are may become the breadcrumbs on your path to discovering the true answer to your puzzle. In the upcoming chapters, we will dive deep into each point of the star so you can clearly pinpoint what you need to shift in order to free yourself from the continual emotional struggle and, as you do that, it will in turn simultaneously move you toward your heart's desire.

I am so excited for you!

I invite you to treat yourself to a pretty, sparkly, colorful notebook or journal to accompany you on this journey. Reading this book won't be a passive activity for entertainment. It will require some work from you. But I promise you the work will be so worth it. There will be thought-provoking questions and prompts, suggestions, reflections, and activities in many of the chapters, and your journal will be a special place for you to capture them. Writing down thoughts and feelings that come up for you will bring greater clarity and will make it easier to determine your missing piece(s).

Your personal discovery through this process and the actions you take to execute what you learn will be what creates positive and lasting change to align your mind, body, and spirit to receiving your baby. That knowledge, coupled with your increasing self-awareness and insights gained that you apply to your personal situation, will be *your magic* in the middle of *your* story, so I do encourage you to be completely open and honest with yourself.

You will notice that I reference God or Jesus at different points throughout the book. I use these words because they are representative of my personal faith walk and Christianity belief system. However, I encourage you to exchange those words, if they don't align with your spiritual beliefs, to ones that do, be it Universe, Source, Nature, Life Force, Higher Power, or something else. That way the concepts being explained using these words will resonate with what you know to be true for you so you can comfortably apply them to your life.

I am 100 percent committed to giving you all that I've got, and I have no doubt that you will do the same for yourself or you wouldn't be reading this book.

I am so excited for this part of your journey. Your life is never going to be the same from this point on.

Let the magic begin!

SECTION ONE
In the Dark

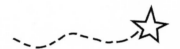

Chapter One
Have You Tried Everything?

What controls your attention controls your life.

—Darren Hardy

My typical modus operandi (m.o.) when I am faced with a challenge, or a significant problem is to become solution focused and tap into my resourcefulness, creativity, and perseverance. I am relentless at figuring things out until I accomplish the goal in front of me. I pride myself on being a good problem solver.

I'm not afraid of hard work, and I like to achieve. I put in the effort, work hard, research my options, brainstorm new ideas, stay motivated, keep trying, and the results I'm looking for come my way. It was a formula I could generally rely on having great success with, except when it came to my infertility.

Not only was my body failing me but also my usual tactics and strategies were coming up short, which made me feel more inadequate. Why wasn't it working? My approach seemed to be a good one. Hadn't I thought of everything? Hadn't I tried everything? I thought I was covering all the bases.

Well, let's look at this together, so the missing piece can be revealed.

My first order of business when I was initially diagnosed with infertility was to do a complete battery of tests to determine any potential physiological causes of it.

Findings:

Dawn—High FSH, low ovarian reserve, and premature menopause predicted.

Tom—Low sperm count, abnormally shaped sperm, and low sperm motility.

Action Taken:

Three unsuccessful IUIs (intrauterine insemination)

One unsuccessful IVF (in vitro fertilization)

My endocrinologist recommended we go the egg-donor route at this point because of my egg-quality issues and that I was already given the highest dose of hormones for IVF and still only barely met the criteria of the required four egg follicles.

As you may recall from what I shared previously, our IVF attempt ended early because the sperm and eggs did not fertilize. My husband felt that with these ART (assisted reproductive technology) procedures, it was like putting our money on a roulette wheel and hoping our number would come up. We decided to put these procedures to rest and continue trying to conceive on our own, despite the extremely poor odds.

One of the strategies I was unfailingly consistent with, and I'm sure you can relate to, was identifying my prime fertility window. Today, there are ovulation tests to make it more convenient, but when I was trying to conceive, I had the assistance of a trusty ovulation symptom chart where I tracked my basal body temperature each day of the month and assessed the color and consistency of my cervical mucous to more clearly identify when ovulation would occur.

I was keenly aware of how long an egg was viable after being released and how long sperm live. Given my husband's sperm issues, we were advised to have intercourse every other day during our fertile window, as opposed to consecutive days, to maximize his sperm concentration.

I bought into the practice of staying flat on my back after intercourse with hips tilted and legs elevated for ten minutes so gravity wasn't working against me, and I was therefore—I believed—assisting the sperm to reach their destination more easily. (The things we do to maximize our chances!)

Speaking of maximizing chances, I recall one evening informing my husband that we needed to have sex that night because it was our prime time for conceiving. He said he was really tired, and that he wanted to save it for the next night.

What?? Save it for tomorrow night like we were a couple who didn't have fertility issues?? We have to maximize our chances to the fullest, I thought as I cried myself to sleep (quietly) wondering if we had just given up the *one* time we might have actually conceived. What if *that* night would have been our time?

People in our position don't have the luxury of doing that.

Driving to the gym the next morning, I reflected on how I felt that night. The lack of control I felt was immense. I can't control my infertility issues. I can't *make* my husband have sex with me. That's out of my control. *How was I ever going to have a baby?* The desperation I sensed was growing out of control too. It's pretty sad when the poor guy isn't allowed to be tired because I feel so forced to utilize every opportunity.

In the midst of the ART procedures, I was working as an elementary school counselor while trying to juggle the many medical appointments and the emotional roller coaster that infertility and treatments generate. My anxiety level was on the rise and the stress that ensued from all of it was impacting my confidence level at work, creating further stress for me. I experienced panic attacks multiple times a day and worried when the next one might happen. I wondered if the amount of stress at work was interfering with getting pregnant, which I wasn't willing to continue. It was time to minimize my life stressors and rule that out as a possible contributor, so I resigned from my position. But even four years after resigning, I still wasn't pregnant.

My mother is a devout Catholic and I was raised to strictly conform to the teachings of Catholicism. St. Gerard is the patron saint of expectant mothers and having a devotion to St. Gerard helps encourage him to intercede for you regarding your infertility. My priest let me borrow a relic of St. Gerard, and I prayed the nine-day Novena several times to him. I kept it displayed on my bedroom dresser and even took it with me to hold during my ART procedures.

Even prior to the onset of our fertility diagnoses, I had been actively involved in two different prayer groups. Strengthening my relationship with God has always been important to me and at that time, I needed Him more than ever. Both prayer groups along with family and friends outside these groups prayed for me to conceive. My prayer warriors were on the job!

I had a daily ritual of declaring specific scriptures out loud to demonstrate my belief in God's promises. Here are a couple examples of the many scriptures I proclaimed:

> *And whatever you ask for in prayer, having faith and (really) believing, you will receive.*
>
> Matthew 21:22

> *Truly I tell you, whoever says to this mountain, be lifted up and thrown into the sea! And does not doubt at all in his heart but believes that what he says will take place, it will be done for him.*
>
> Mark 11:23

That *mountain* in my case referred to my infertility.

My prayer warriors emphasized strongly, "When you say these scriptures, you must believe—truly believe—it will come to pass and thank God that it has already been done."

I would say with conviction, "I do believe."

I believed because my faith in God was strong. I had witnessed God do amazing things in my life before in answer to prayer, and I knew that since God put this strong desire in my heart to have a baby, then surely, He would answer this prayer too in the way I wanted. I had faith, trust, and confidence in Him and that He wouldn't let me down.

Yes, I believed, but did I believe without any doubt?

During this time, my sister was being treated by a naturopathic practitioner for multiple sclerosis. During one of her visits, my sister shared our infertility struggle, and this naturopath recommended that my husband and I both be evaluated by her and begin a wellness program individualized to meet our specific needs. She claimed this would get our bodies in optimal health, condition, and balance to create the most hospitable environment for conception to occur. She stated that she had helped every infertile couple in her program to conceive through her treatment regimen. This made perfect sense and offered a lot of hope.

The wellness program was intense and quite the commitment in many ways. We traveled over four hours round trip once or more a month for what ended up being a total of three years. It was challenging to adhere to the strict guidelines and be so disciplined. We were permitted to eat only organic foods, and we had to eliminate red meat, dairy, white flour, sugar, alcohol, caffeine, and processed foods completely from our diet. We needed to be sure our daily water intake was equivalent to half of our body weight in ounces. We were on a strict regimen of supplements, probiotics, vitamins, and homeopathics that were individualized to each of our body's needs. We were each on a specific daily dosing schedule multiple times a day in a certain order and had parameters for ingesting them that had to be followed. It was a lot of change all at one time.

We made lifestyle changes to minimize the amount of toxicity we were absorbing into our bodies via computer usage, cell phones, and microwave usage. Of course, regular exercise was a must, but thankfully we already had that piece in place.

We were the healthiest we had ever been. My irritable bowel syndrome (IBS) symptoms that I suffered with daily for years significantly improved. I was doing my body good!

But I was STILL. NOT. PREGNANT!

Dori, our naturopath, was stumped as well and thought there may likely be an emotional component interfering with conception. How right she was and pinpointing and addressing it just might have done the trick, which is what we are going to do for you with the content of this book.

Next in line to try was acupuncture. Through my research to understand and reverse my infertility, I discovered that acupuncture helps to regulate hormone function and increase blood flow to the uterus and ovaries making it easier to conceive. Acupuncture also lowers stress levels, which we know is key to fertility.

We found a local certified acupuncturist, and my husband and I both received acupuncture treatments regularly for a year.

Needles galore.

Still, no baby.

Oh, and let's not forget my almost daily obsession of scavenging the internet for the latest supplement, technique, and known belief that claimed to increase chances of conception. I had to be sure I wasn't missing anything. Being thorough, determined, and persistent had always worked in my favor.

So, it seems like I covered all the bases, right?

- ☑ Tests to determine any underlying physiological causes of infertility

- ☑ Assisted Reproductive Technology (ART) Procedures— IUI, IVF

- ☑ Maximizing my prime fertility window

- ☑ Quit job to reduce stress level

- ☑ Prayers and steadfast faith

☑ Wellness program to the max including diet, exercise, and holistic approach

☑ Acupuncture

☑ Researched tips/new items on the market to enhance conception

What was I missing? I was doing it all.

That's right. I was *doing, doing, doing*. All on my own agenda. All in the name of trying to make this baby happen. I was on a mission. Fertility, unfortunately, is contrary to the hustle work ethic. It flourishes when there is no forcing, strenuous effort, or urgency.

Getting pregnant is something that just happens. Just like with sleep. You can't "do" sleep. And often the harder you try to make yourself sleep, the more it doesn't happen and the more frustrated you become.

You *fall* asleep. It happens when your mind and body relax. When we create a relaxed environment for sleep to happen, it works in our favor. A baby needs this relaxed environment as well. I was giving it everything but that.

However, when we truly cast our care (worry) to God, we *can* relax. In fact, we do it so we can relax and have peace of mind.

Isn't that what I did with all my prayers and daily rituals of scripture proclaiming?

Not really. It's time to revisit that point I made earlier about believing without any doubt.

Here's the thing. Before you can truly cast your care, you must decide on the front end that you are going to be satisfied with whatever God's answer is because you *know* that no matter what happens, He will work it out for your good, even if it doesn't feel good in the moment. That's a lot of trust. And trust is difficult because we don't always immediately receive what we ask for.

If I'm being completely honest with myself and with you, I wasn't able to surrender to God 100 percent. I wanted to, but my fear was bigger than my faith, I'm sad to say. I was so fearful that God's answer might be no, and that I wouldn't conceive my own baby.

That fear drove all my decisions and my mindset.

Not trust.

I was fearful that if I wasn't trying to control the outcome I wanted when I wanted it (and be in the driver's seat), then I wouldn't get what I wanted.

What's so ironic and ridiculous is that by doing it my way and trying to control everything, I was getting a *no* every time anyway. I was fearful the answer wouldn't be what *I wanted* and the one I *knew* was best for me. I didn't trust that God was working things out for my highest good and that I would be taken care of.

Trust equals confidence. And I wasn't feeling confident I would get a *yes* to a baby.

God was waiting for me to prove that I trusted Him. Not just with my words (scriptures and prayers), but with my deeds (emotions, actions, and behaviors). My words and actions weren't aligned. If they were, I believe His promise would have been fulfilled. We receive from God through faith and patience. He was testing my faith.

This was one of my lessons to learn and perhaps it is yours too. My lesson was to stop relying only on myself and to lean on God. I needed to stop controlling and trying to manipulate the outcome I wanted and was so attached to—the same outcome I was determined *must* be, instead of surrendering to God's knowing with complete abandon. It was a lesson in trust that I failed. And these same lessons in life keep getting presented to us until we learn them.

I now know the message my infertility was trying to send me. It was an opportunity to learn this lesson that would serve me well in my life over and over again. God had to use something of great meaning to me that was so close to my heart, like my passion to become a mother, so it would drive home the lesson He wanted me to learn.

God wasn't saying no to me. He was saying not yet. Oh, but I thought I had to do things my way and not His. I went from one thing to the next in an effort to make this baby happen. I had to be in control because that felt certain and safe to me. Surrender is the unknown, and the unknown feels *un*certain. It felt so scary to let go into the unknown and uncertainty. In my mind at that time, controlling kept me certain. But, certain of what? I believe I felt like I was at least moving in the direction of having a baby with my concerted efforts, rather than just waiting around hoping it would happen.

Control isn't surrender. It's the opposite of surrender. It put me out of alignment because the control was driven by my fear.

My fear was driven by my belief system (that I *needed* to be a mom to feel complete and happy in life). The fear generated by that belief system kept me from being able to surrender.

And fear (which is the stress response) is a dense, heavy energy, the lowest energy frequency, which is not at all conducive to conception. All that trying so hard to fix my situation, improve it, change it, and make this baby happen was just making me spin my wheels. I was exhausting myself with frustration over something of which I had no control. That energy could have been so much more wisely spent.

The funny thing is, we tend to receive what we desire when we don't *need* it so desperately. The heavy energy level of desperation is in opposition to relaxation, contentment, peace, and harmony, which is light. When you are holding on tightly, wanting something so much, you are, in essence, pushing it away further. That resistance deepens and lengthens your pain while keeping the good thing you seek further out of reach. Infertility is painful on many levels, but I created my own suffering by not surrendering. I actually did have control over the amount of pain and suffering I experienced. I just didn't see that back then. I hope you can see this and apply it to your situation if it's applicable.

Not only was I needing to let go and trust God, but I also needed to let go of thinking that I alone could make things happen if I tried hard enough and I *willed* it to be. I was used to making things happen. Try harder, do more, persist, don't give up. I had to let go of this old pattern and this identity of myself. It was time to release my old ways that weren't working anymore. God allows situations to occur to draw us closer to Him so He can be there for us. God doesn't cause our problems. He is the solution to them. If everything went our way all the time, how often do you think we would seek Him? It's the trying times that put us on our knees that test and strengthen our faith.

If we thank God for all those miracles and good things that He seemingly has put in our way, then we still need to have that same faith in Him to come through for us in our pain, loss, tragedy, or outcomes that go differently than we had planned. He is the same God.

I truly think I believed that if I did all these things that I was doing my part and showing God how passionate I was to become a mother. I was fooling myself. I would go on to the next potential solution because I was so scared that I wouldn't become a mother otherwise. I never stopped. I actually believed that my controlling and contorting things was really going to seal the deal.

Let's face it. Conception isn't something we *do* have control over. It requires trust.

Who is going to make that sperm and egg fertilize? GOD!!

Who??

GOD!!

The spark that ignites the start of life is *all* God. He decides.

We really never had control over it anyway; therefore, we haven't *lost* control because of being diagnosed with our infertility. Doctors came up with the magical time frame of one year of trying unsuccessfully before being concerned if you're not pregnant. What if it was typical for it to take three years before being concerned? People wouldn't panic so soon and maybe not get into stress mode until then.

My point is that we need to not let medical time frames and, in my case, a 2 percent chance of getting pregnant discourage us and decide our destiny, otherwise we become victims. It's what we tell ourselves about the diagnosis and prognosis that stresses us and exacerbates the problem. What we focus on magnifies, so we need to have thoughts aligned with the outcome we desire. Keep in mind, statistics are general and not personal. You could be in the small percentage of success. Why not? Someone is, why not you? You can't limit your thinking.

So, what *would* proving I trusted God have looked like?

A trusting mama-to-be wouldn't have been in such a frenzied, worried, and controlling state. She would be in the present moment enjoying her life to the fullest, being grateful for what she *does* have right in front of her. She would make love to her husband genuinely in response to her love for him, not controlling it, manipulating it, and forcing it to happen based on an ovulation schedule. She would do this because she trusts that God can do *all* things, schedule or no schedule.

A trusting mama-to-be would have been grateful to take part in that holistic wellness program, knowing she was doing the utmost for her health to create an optimum environment for her baby to develop when the time came, but I begrudgingly partook in that wellness program. I was resentful that I had to give up so much and do so much that so many other women didn't have to do to become pregnant. My intention behind that wellness program didn't come from my soul, but from my ego. My fear drove me to do it, emanating a low energy frequency of resentment, jealousy, and injustice. Not a match for manifesting a baby. It was doomed from the start.

A surrendered mama-to-be wouldn't comb the internet daily to look for more solutions and obsessively check and re-check pregnancy symptoms online hoping that *this* time she was experiencing implantation symptoms and not premenstrual ones. She wouldn't feel the need to do that because she would feel free and relaxed in her trust in God. She would know that if God didn't answer her prayer in the way she would like, it's because He had something better planned for her. I needed less Google and more God!

Had I behaved like a trusting—believing without a doubt—surrendered mama wannabe and waited for God's nudges for my next steps on my journey (instead of taking them into my own hands out of desperation), God would have witnessed my unwavering faith and fulfilled the promise of His word according to scriptures.

I was my own worst enemy.

So, I implore you to garner wisdom from my experience and take very seriously this act of surrender. I needed to have someone sit me down, look me straight in the eyes, and say, "Dawn, your emotional state and behavior are not evidence of someone who believes, trusts, and knows that God will come through for you. You are getting in your own way."

Let *me* be that person for you. Let me help you surrender, find your inner peace, and enjoy your present life as it is now while you continue on your way to becoming the mother you desire to be.

⸙——Reflections and Journal Prompts

What bases have you covered so far?

Do you lean on a higher power for guidance, strength, wisdom, and comfort?

Who is in the driver's seat most of the time?

Chapter Two
Stress

Until you make the unconscious conscious, it will direct your life and you will call it fate.

—C. G. Jung

Before we delve into the Five-Point SuperStar System, let's talk about stress first.

How many times has someone said to you in reference to your infertility, "You just need to relax, then it will happen?"

For me, too many to count.

That very comment alone would increase my stress level on the spot because, even if I didn't come back with a verbal response, I felt defensive internally for several reasons.

> **One**, *you* try relaxing when you have tried to get pregnant for consecutive years and it's the one thing you want more

than anything in the world. *And* your biological clock is quickly ticking since you are already in your early forties.

Two, there are real biological reasons as to why I am struggling to conceive—My low egg reserve and poor egg quality and my husband's low sperm count and poor sperm quality.

Three, that comment always made me feel like I alone was responsible for my infertility issues, like I was the cause of them and that it could just turn around on a dime if I would just get my act together, calm down, and relax.

I know the *just relax* comments didn't have any ill intent behind them and that the people saying them probably believed they were being helpful. But it made me angry because they didn't understand how incredibly challenging struggling with this condition is and their seemingly cavalier comment, as if it's easy to fix, basically confirmed that for me.

I think my defensiveness stemmed from feeling like I was being criticized for something that wasn't my fault or within my control. What's interesting though is that my defensiveness didn't allow me to look for any truth in that comment.

If so many people were saying this to me, could they *all* be wrong? Was it really that they just didn't understand and wanted to say a flippant comment *or* was the stress I was under truly getting in the way?

I couldn't see it back then. I was so hell-bent on defending my victimhood and consumed by emotion that I was unable to step back and see the many ways I was contributing to my own suffering and in turn making conception less likely to occur.

Now, don't get me wrong, infertility in and of itself is very stressful. Researchers from *Evie Magazine* state that the levels of anxiety and depression experienced by those diagnosed with infertility is comparable to patients diagnosed with cancer, HIV, and heart disease (Gallagher, December 15, 2021). However, I took that stress to a whole new level of suffering by engaging in mindsets and behaviors that didn't serve me well and by *not* engaging in those that would. More than likely, you have been doing the same thing, especially if you feel like you are at an emotional breaking point.

I have come to realize that these unhelpful mindsets and behaviors were most likely the culprit that blocked me from conceiving, further perpetuating my infertility. I know this may sound like a stretch but stay with me here: It may have initially even set me up to be infertile because of the toll chronic patterns of poor stress management and living inauthentically can have on the body.

Well, that's a tough pill to swallow now, isn't it?!

I don't bring this up to play the blame game and make you—or myself for that matter—feel that we *caused* our infertility, or we are the reason we are struggling to conceive, but rather to take ownership of the role we *do* play, even if it's indirectly. You can't blame yourself for something you weren't aware could be having such a profound impact.

So, no blame here.

When you have awareness, you can take responsibility. When you take responsibility, you can make change happen that can get you what you want. Then, *you* have the power instead of allowing this infertility to have power over you. Now, that's something to celebrate! If limiting, negative belief patterns and subsequent emotions can cause so much trouble, just think what rectifying this can do for overall wellbeing and quality of life. Then, we aren't at the mercy of chance or just bad luck; we have much more control over our bodies and our lives than we ever anticipated. That's very liberating.

You *can* turn this around! This *is* fixable! This is exciting news! I hope you see it and you haven't allowed your ego to get in the way and become defensive to what I've just shared. Stay open. Being open is a key ingredient to getting pregnant.

How Stress Affects Your Body

Our nervous system goes into alarm mode of fight or flight when we are under stress. It is hardwired to mobilize resources and deprioritize any systems of the body not necessary for immediate survival, such as digestion, elimination, our higher brain centers, and reproduction, so energy can be conserved for that purpose. Our immune system is compromised as well. Back in primitive times, this survival mode went into action to defend us from a saber-toothed tiger. This was great, because we needed 100 percent of our energy put into our muscles to save our life. The problem is, these days that same stress response still happens; now it is not with a tiger, but with our boss, our husband, our finances, or infertility.

Infertility is considered a disease of the reproductive system. Merriam-Webster defines *disease* as a condition that prevents the body or mind from working normally. Thankfully, infertility is not life-threatening, but it still constitutes a disease. Experts say the fundamental cause of disease is stress.

Chronic disease, which develops over time, is best treated by looking at the whole individual: mind and body and spirit. It has been my experience that the medical field generally only addresses the physical body when it comes to infertility. It is my intent, through the attention this book receives and the success stories of women like you embracing treating your infertility with mind, body, and spirit, that this holistic approach to treating infertility will become the norm. This approach could serve as a proactive measure that ob-gyn practices use and make available as standard protocol to their patients who desire to have children, so perhaps infertility diagnoses could significantly decline.

As you can see, being in a chronic state of stress is counter-productive to getting pregnant. Our bodies are wise and know when it's a safe or unsafe time to procreate.

You may be thinking, *Well, this is all well and good Dawn, but how can I not be stressed?? I can't get pregnant/stay pregnant? This is stressful!*

You are right, it certainly is. However, staying in a stressed state won't get you what you want. We are going to get down to the nitty-gritty and get specific on what you need to shift so that you are aligned mind, body, and spirit to allow this beautiful miracle of life to grow in you.

Fear, doubt, worry, and anxiety are all low frequency energy levels, and we attract what we put out in terms of energy. When we want to attract abundance into our lives (and a baby to love is the utmost in abundance), we need to regularly be in an emotional state that matches that. That congruent energy frequency is peace, joy, love, and harmony. This doesn't mean that it's not okay to feel the full range of emotion—and you certainly will because that is part of the human experience—but your dominant emotion will need to be one that supports your living your best life and I know for you that includes being a mom.

The challenge is getting yourself to be there while coping with your infertility. That's where the tools come in that I'm going to show you. Incorporating these into your life will assist you in keeping your state (emotions/energy/frequency level) at a place that maintains your alignment (feeling balanced, calm, and centered), therefore attracting that which brings joy, peace, and love into your life.

These tools are simple in concept but not always easy to do because they require you to be conscious of your thoughts, feelings, beliefs, and actions. So many of us go about our day on autopilot and typically just react to situations we are presented with rather than consciously choosing our thoughts and actions to create the outcomes we desire. If you put in the effort, you will most certainly reap the reward.

The beautiful thing is that by making these lifestyle changes you will not only feel a whole lot better emotionally, but you will also acquire a level of self-mastery that will benefit you in overcoming your infertility and be able to carry with you in all areas of your life from here on out. You have nothing to lose and so much to gain.

Imagine this scale as you are learning these tools throughout the following chapters.

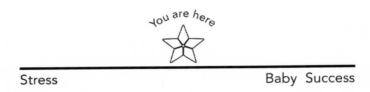

Stress   Baby Success

For discussion purposes, let's say you are smack in the middle of this scale where the star marks the spot. To your right is your destination, your goal, where you plan to arrive. To your left is misery—more misery and suffering. Based on how you have been feeling lately, you may determine that your star should be placed closer to the left of where I placed it, or even perhaps all the way to the far left. You make that call for yourself because only you know.

As you learn the valuable tools and begin to recognize your typical patterns of thinking and behaving, you will be able to assess whether what you are doing is moving you toward your baby or whether it is moving you away from it and increasing your stress level. Then you can course correct as needed. This will be an insightful and practical tool to keep you conscious and empowered on your journey to motherhood.

Please be assured that the intent behind using this tool is not to make you paranoid of every move you make or cause you to convict and judge yourself, but merely to increase self-awareness and encourage self-growth.

So, let's get you out of survival mode and into procreation mode!

Shift Your Belief About Stress

One of the first steps I'd like you to take is changing how you view stress. Yes, stress is uncomfortable and can negatively impact our bodies, but it is also our feedback system. The changes we experience in our bodies are there to alert us that we aren't physiologically and psychologically in equilibrium and things are awry. It's a warning to do what we need to do to reestablish homeostasis. We can choose to view it as a huge wake-up call about poor habits we may have had for years and make the necessary changes, or we can continue down our same path not heeding the warning and pay a price for it. It's our choice.

The body and mind are so connected. We can create reactions in our bodies from our thoughts alone. Our thoughts can make us sick, or they can help heal us. That's how powerful they are.

Here's a quick example.

I don't like to fly in an airplane. Turbulence scares me because I don't know when it's going to stop and restart or if it means we may have an accident, and generally because I feel out of control when it's happening. I also get horrible pain in my inner ear as a result of the air pressure changes when the plane descends. I wear ear plugs designed to address this issue, but it's not a perfect fix. So, needless to say, I dread flying but desire to go the places the plane can take me.

If I think about all the reasons I don't like flying while I am on the plane or even prior to boarding, I will feel physical reactions to those anxiety-provoking thoughts. My heart rate will rise, my breathing will get shallow, I'll start to feel nauseous, light-headed, and my IBS symptoms may even kick in. Not very pleasant.

However, if I focus my thoughts on what I *can* do to make the most of the flight and say to myself,

> *Now, I have a chance to read that book I have been wanting to.*

> *In two hours, I'll be in sunny Florida, soon to be on a beach.*

> *And, if turbulence does arise, flight attendants tell me there have not been any plane crashes as a result of turbulence. It's just bumps in the air like bumps in the road when I'm driving.*

When I have *these* thoughts, I feel more at peace and calmer without the physical reactions I mentioned earlier. *I control* how my body responds based on *my thoughts*. We *think* we have no control over our bodies and that they just do what they are going to do. That's a false belief.

So, if you start to view stress through the lens of it being your partner/friend instead of your enemy because it is your feedback mechanism indicating you are out of alignment, and as a result, you feel gratitude for it, it can actually help to regulate your stress response. Pretty cool, right? This small shift in thinking gives you a huge payoff.

Be conscious of your body and catch your "friend's" signal early so it can allow you to get curious and intentionally make positive changes to better manage your stressors.

What are *your* signs of stress?

☐ Increased heartrate

☐ Muscle tension (where do you feel it?)

☐ Shoulders up to your ears

☐ Sweating

☐ Headaches

☐ Nausea

☐ Bowel trouble

☐ Depression

☐ Frequent sickness

☐ Skin issues

☐ Chronic pain

☐ Insomnia

☐ Fatigue

☐ Numbing or distracting yourself from emotional pain with any of the following: social media, busyness, alcohol, TV binge watching, overworking, online shopping, overeating/indulging in sugar/junk food

☐ Or something else?

Thank your body for this information and then dig deeper into what it's trying to tell you needs to change.

❤ Reflections and Journal Prompts

How does stress show up for you? What physical symptoms do you experience? Emotional symptoms? What behaviors do you engage in?

What do you think your infertility is trying to tell you? What message is it sending you?

You may not be ready or able to answer this right now, but asking the questions leaves you open to receive the answers. Be compassionate and patient with yourself.

If you don't feel ready, ask yourself why. Why don't I feel ready? I don't feel ready because_____. This answer is also important information for you. What is your resistance (unreadiness) saying?

SECTION TWO
The Five-Point
SuperStar System

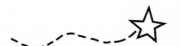

Chapter Three
Surrender

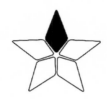

The beginning of anxiety is the end of faith, and
the beginning of faith is the end of anxiety.

—George Mueller

Surrender is the first of the five points of the SuperStar System.
There are many misconceptions about what it means to surrender.
It can often have a negative connotation as in losing or giving up or
giving in. In this chapter, you will get clarity on what it really means
to surrender and how it can be a positive and empowering force in
your life, particularly when it comes to your infertility. Let's talk
about some key concepts of surrender and ways to assist you in
doing it.

God Is Working for You, Not Against You

God gave you this strong, passionate desire in your heart to become
a mother and have a baby. God is pure love. A baby is love. This

desire comes from love. A mother's love is profound. God wants you to receive this desire of your heart because He put it on your heart. Believe that without a doubt. You wouldn't have been given the desire if you weren't given the ability to fulfill it. You are equipped for it. Trust that God knows all, and His timing of this and the way in which it unfolds in your life will be for your highest good.

You must have this belief to be able to completely surrender. Then, there will be no fear. You will operate from love and not fear. The energy of fear and what it does to the body keeps your baby away from you. And it affirms your lack of trust. You co-create with God when you are aligned with Him, while fear and doubt knock you out of alignment with God. Love, the ultimate and high-level energy frequency, will bring your baby to you. Remembering God's love for you and believing that He will do what is best for you will enhance your trust.

Surrender Is Letting Go and Taking Responsibility

Recognize that surrender doesn't mean you are giving up on your goal. You are creating space for it to happen. It opens you up and frees you to receive. You are then open to conceive. You are telling God that you are ready, you trust Him completely, you have let go of your ways, and you are open to receiving your highest good because only He knows that best. God always has your highest good and best interest in His thoughts and plans for you, even if you can't see it in your present circumstances. Gripping or holding on for dear life is blocking your blessing.

Casting your care and surrendering doesn't mean you sit back passively and do nothing. Surrender also doesn't mean that you give up what you want, but that you stop dictating how it all needs to happen. You allow and trust God to help *you do your best* in the situation and let God do the rest.

Surrender Requires Trust

Trust is having confidence. Confidence is a feeling or a belief that one can rely on someone or something. You are certain of its truth. Although I had trust in God based on what I had seen Him do in my life before, I still struggled with trusting Him completely with this baby thing. We can't really be sure of the level of trust we have in God until it is put to the test, and we are certainly put to the test with the infertility struggle.

It is not only imperative that you believe God always has your highest good in mind and will answer your prayer if it's according to His will, but also that if He doesn't give you it, it's because it's not time yet or He has something better planned for you. My challenge came with part two of that belief. I struggled with trying to reason with *What could be better for me than having my own baby?*

I mean really! What could be better for me than that, given it's all I thought about and wanted since I was little? Well, if I really wanted to *know* what could be better, I guess I'd have to surrender to find out. I didn't want to believe that my *not* having my own baby could be in my highest good. That mindset kept me—instead of Jesus—in control and in the driver's seat. I wanted to do everything in my power to get pregnant. I wasn't taking God's lead. I was bossing Him around, trying to get Him to do things my way. It's like a sick person going to the doctor for help but then dictating what the doctor should do to cure the person. *What?* No wonder I didn't feel at peace. No wonder I kept hitting walls and closed doors at every turn. None of us will feel inner peace trying to make something happen that only God can do.

All God was waiting for was my trust. So interesting. The root cause of not being able to surrender is the fear that we won't get what we want unless we take care of it ourselves. Yep, that was me. Usually surrendering is the *last* course of action people take once they have exhausted themselves and are fed up with being miserable. Let it be your *first* course of action. Real trust yields good fruit. This trust and the peace that ensues as a result of it prompts God to work on our behalf to invoke justice in our circumstance.

Surrendering really *would* have been doing everything in my power to have a baby because it would have yielded the results I wanted, unlike the stress and resistance I was encountering from *not* surrendering (which was counterproductive to my many efforts anyway). I was a control freak and an anxious madwoman when, instead, I could have been coasting along, riding free in the peace of trusting God, and resting in the knowing of His highest good for me.

Here's the truth in a nutshell. We need to want what *God wants* for us because then we can't lose. If it ends up *not* being what we want, we know it will be even better for us. Yes, I wanted to be a mom and God wanted that for me too. He wanted me to trust Him to do it His way and in His timing. If I had done that, I would have had peace during my wait. If I didn't do that, I would suffer and keep postponing receiving what I was praying for. There you have it. It was up to me.

At one point, I even started praying to God that He would take away my desire to want to have a baby. I was all over the place! If I couldn't have this baby, then I was begging to *not want one*. It felt like a cruel joke. My emotional pain resulting from desiring something so much and having seemingly no control over getting it to happen was so unbearable to me. I felt it was better for God to just remove the desire from my heart if He wasn't going to say yes to my conceiving. That was my plan for resolving my excruciating pain and inner turmoil. Talk about being in a frenzied state!! Talk about me proving that I didn't trust Him. He was probably just shaking his head at me, hoping I would get it soon.

God heard my prayer but didn't respond as I anticipated. My desire to be a mother to such a strong degree was gifted to me from God and part of His plan for my highest good. So, He wasn't about to remove it. The thing is, we aren't privy to the BIG picture, the long-range grander plan. Only God has that knowledge, which is where trust comes in. We can't see in our present circumstances how this experience will fit into the BIG plan He has in store for us or how it will all be worked out for our highest good. He knows what our soul needs on our journey to become the best versions of ourselves in this lifetime. Our prayers are answered in proportion to our level of spiritual maturity. Sometimes God needs to prepare us in specific ways before we can receive our blessing. Or sometimes it's other people, in relation to that circumstance, who need to be prepared, which can delay the manifestation of it in our lives. God knows how all things work intricately together for the highest good, yet we, however, don't—in that moment anyway. But, if we hold on to the belief that He does, trusting in Him becomes easier.

Oh, how I wish I would have trusted. I did *eventually* trust and surrender but getting this earlier would have saved me a lot of unnecessary suffering. Now that I have more of the BIG picture than I did back then, it is very clear to me why God did things in the manner that He did. I can assure you that God makes good come from the pain we feel in the unjust circumstances in our life if we maintain a good attitude while going through it. Faith is always accompanied by a good attitude for it to *be* faith. I will offer you my understanding of this toward the end of the book when I share specifically how God chose to answer my prayer to become a mother.

God is our father, and we are His children. And just like a parent with their child, we don't give them everything that they want exactly when they want it. Sometimes a child needs to hear no or not right now without any explanation other than that the parent knows what is best for them. Sometimes it is about things they wouldn't understand at their level of development, and they just need to trust that the parent is wiser and sees the big picture for their own good. Sometimes, it's good to not get what we want right away. There are lessons in that. This is the same with God.

Being able to trust God and have confidence in knowing that He always has your back will allow you to experience peace in your mind, body, and soul. This will enable you to enjoy your life to the fullest.

Trust enables you to give your mind a rest from ruminating and trying to figure things out. My mind was always on overdrive, clearly indicating I wasn't trusting. Our challenging experiences in life help us to grow our trust. You need to *experience* what trusting can do for you. No one can do it for you. Our trust grows in times of trial like this because without trials and tribulations in our lives, we wouldn't have a need to seek God and put Him first. It's how God reveals to us where we need to grow to become more like Him. Then, we can take this earned wisdom and spiritual growth from our experience with trust and apply the learning to trials down the road. Our trials ground us in our faith.

If you reflect on your own level of trust as you read this and recognize that your trust is lacking, be honest with yourself and God. He already knows anyway. Ask him to strengthen your trust so that you can surrender. It's a process and we are all at different stages. Sometimes we surrender and then we slip up, requiring us to surrender again and again. It's okay. We are human. The humility in seeking God's help with this will be most pleasing to Him and He will come through for you. So, don't let a lack of trust keep you from surrendering.

Surrender Is Freedom

There are some things we *can* control in life. We can control our thoughts, the words we speak, the actions we take, the level of effort we put forth toward something, the meaning we give to things, our response to situations, or how we show up in life (our attitude)— basically, everything which emanates from within us and is within this present moment from which we make our decisions. This is our power to influence what happens in our lives. However, we don't have direct control over the outcomes in our lives—what is external to us. We may be able to influence them, but we can't control or force them. This is why we can get so frustrated, disappointed, and depressed trying to control what we are unable to control. So, when I am speaking about control relative to surrender, I am referring to our outcomes, such as the outcome of conceiving a baby or not. It is an outcome and something we don't have control over. We can certainly influence it with the right mindset, decisions, actions, and emotions, but whether it occurs or not is out of our hands. And our journey to that outcome will certainly be more pleasant with positive influences and a high energy level.

Control (being controlling and trying to control or force) is the opposite of surrender. We control out of fear and our need to know or be certain. When we surrender, we let go into something beyond our known ideas, beyond what we can conceive in our minds. Needing to know is restrictive because with our limited minds, we can only conjure up a finite number of possibilities regarding our circumstances. God has infinite possibilities, and remember, He has the BIG picture in mind, which is expansive.

Control is constrictive. Closed. Limiting.

Surrender is expansive. Open. Limitless.

Control is being resistant to what *is*. It's fighting against the current and not being in flow. This is exhausting and is often counterproductive. It definitely was both of those for me. Surrender means letting go of trying to force life to be a particular way. The desire for things to be different than they are creates stress and suffering within us. We have an attachment to a particular outcome. The attachment is the expectation. When the outcome is different from expectation, we resort to controlling things to meet that expectation instead of surrendering to what is.

This reminds me of a time when I was on vacation with a couple of my girlfriends celebrating my birthday. We were in Puerto Vallarta and had booked a boat excursion to a private island that included dinner and a show. I had heard the ocean water could be rough enough that some guests would get seasick, so I made sure I took Dramamine ahead of time. Once our boat started to get out into the main water at full speed, I could feel the rocking and started to panic and feel queasy in anticipation of feeling like this for the hour-long boat ride with no escape. The more I started to panic, the worse things seemed to be. I certainly wasn't enjoying the moment with my friends on the water.

I said to my girlfriend Dena, "I don't like this."

She could see the fear in my eyes and said, "Dawn, just move your hips with the rhythm of the waves. Breathe deeply. Join in the rocking motion. Go with it. Don't resist it."

As soon as I did that, it was magical. I was in flow with the boat on the water. I felt relaxed. My fear dissipated, and I enjoyed the ride. I surrendered to the rocking waters and allowed it to be instead of fighting against it.

That is very freeing. Resisting wasn't going to change it. It only made me miserable. Once I surrendered, peace came upon me, and I enjoyed the experience.

This is similar to our infertility journey. I didn't like that I was diagnosed with infertility (just like I didn't like the strong waves) and that I had to struggle so much with what seemed to come easily for so many others. It was unacceptable to me. My *expectation* was to conceive babies, and I was very attached to that. My resistance of a different reality than I expected brought on fear, need for control, and the fact that I was fighting every step of the way for it to be *different than it was*. All of this made me miserable, stressed, anxious, and it made life difficult to enjoy. This put me in a state that wasn't conducive to conception. I was trying to force life to be a certain way—my way.

It's so much more freeing to not hold on so tightly to *your* way—how you think it *has* to turn out, how you need it to look, to be, to happen. It's certainly not fun, all that manipulating. It's not easy or enjoyable because you are out of alignment when you do this. The emotional pain and anguish you feel as a result is the indicator that this is the case. Whenever you don't feel good, you aren't in alignment. Everything we do has a tradeoff of some sort. I wanted to remain in control. I didn't want to let go and trust. I wanted to do it my way. My tradeoff to have *that* was giving up peace and instead I was stressed, anxious, and frustrated. To *have* that control, you give up peace. To choose surrender, you give up certainty. But remember, *control* is just a concept in our minds because we can't control our outcomes. We don't gain anything positive with that choice. With surrender, we think we give up certainty, but our certainty will shift in perception. Your trust in God gives you confidence which is its own certainty you can rest in.

Surrender means you aren't attached to a particular outcome. When you surrender, you are open to what God is seeking to have happen in your life, and this is better than what you could ever imagine!

Serenity Prayer

*God grant me the serenity
to accept the things I cannot change,
The courage to change the things I can,
And the wisdom to know the difference.*

Surrender Isn't Automatic Just Because There Is Acceptance

When we accept something, we believe and recognize the reality of what is. We don't have to like it to accept it. We realize the truth of it. Once we accept something, we are then in position to take next steps from that place of acceptance. However, we can be in acceptance but still not surrender.

Let's use the beginning of the COVID-19 pandemic as an example. We had to accept the reality of the shutdown and being confined to our homes except for necessities. That was our reality. Accepting it, but not surrendering to it, would be fighting against it by moaning and groaning with negativity because it was not the experience we thought we should be having. In essence, we were allowing the situation to control our level of happiness. Surrendering would be yielding to it and participating with it without struggle. In this case, we would be open to what was happening. It still didn't mean we liked it, but we made the most of what was. Surrender is content acceptance instead of pissed off/angry acceptance. Let's call it acceptance with a smile.

Surrender is such a powerful thing. I have read that a thousand prayers cannot equal a single act of surrender. God performs His works in proportion to the level of our surrender. Read that sentence again. The degree to which you surrender has a direct effect on the quality of your life.

When our level of happiness is contingent upon whether things go the way we want them to, we are then at the mercy of being batted around emotionally by our circumstances. Getting to the point in our lives where we can be content, emotionally regulated, stable and constant, regardless of and despite our circumstances, is truly empowering. It is one of the best lessons and secrets of life to become skilled in.

Doing the work in this book and applying it in your life consistently will assist you in getting to that place. That is true freedom.

Surrender Requires Facing Your Fears

You can't truly surrender until you address your fears. It's hard to let go when you are fearful of something. The fears stem from limiting beliefs. A whole chapter in this book is devoted to this area, so dig deep into this for yourself. For now, consider this: What is the worst-case scenario that you can conjure up in your mind that could happen if you would relinquish your control and surrender completely to God's will and plan for you?

Really take some time to reflect on this. Be completely honest with yourself. The fear is something to be understood. Dissect it. It's showing you what needs to be worked on within yourself so your desire can manifest.

Then, be with that worst-case scenario. Feel all the feelings. Cry, scream, get angry, and grieve it. Whatever it takes to let the emotions move through you, endure it. Don't judge them. Be compassionate with yourself. They aren't good or bad. They just are. Surrender to these feelings so the fear doesn't have power over you anymore, and you can allow yourself to fully surrender. Once you acknowledge the worst-case scenario, become comfortable with it, and come to terms with it, it frees you up because it no longer has a hold over you. Facing the fear instead of avoiding it diminishes the power it holds.

My worst-case scenario: Who was Dawn if she wasn't a mother? Becoming a mother had become part of my identity. Everything else I had done career-wise was a means to an end until I could eventually get to my true love and passion—motherhood. I perceived my value and worthiness to be wrapped up in this role.

Surrender Is Presence

Surrender removes anxiety because you are fully trusting God with your circumstance. Anxiety arises from thinking about the past or worrying about the future. As soon as we move into worrying, we aren't trusting God. Surrender allows you to be in the present moment and accept what is. Being present allows you to experience peace and be in alignment, which creates ideal fertile ground. Surrender is one of the greatest gifts you can give yourself.

Surrender also reinforces hope. Hope is holding the expectation with certainty that something good is going to happen to you at any moment. You may not know or be certain of how the outcome is going to look or come about, but you know it will be great and in your highest good. Trust is a belief, a knowing deep within your soul.

Believe to receive and conceive.

Surrender Minimizes Self-Absorption

When we are focused on our problem, our situation—how to fix it, how to manage it, and how it makes us feel—it means we have ourselves on our minds a lot. We become self-absorbed. It takes up a lot of our time and attention. I know for me, trying to become pregnant was consuming my life. My mind was focused on making everything about me—what I didn't have, what I was missing out on, what I wasn't being blessed with. No wonder I felt so horrible. It took so much of my energy trying to figure things out all the time. Too much of anything isn't a good thing. It's out of balance and it puts us out of balance.

When you surrender and put your trust in God, it frees you from needing to do it all. The pressure you put on yourself to figure this out disappears, and you and your circumstance aren't on your mind all the time. God would rather see us helping others with their problems than focusing so much on ourselves. And, when we do this, we are sowing good seed.

When we take our eyes off ourselves and seek to be a blessing to others, our blessing finds us. Look to make a difference in someone else's life. Think about who in your life could use an encouraging word, a favor, or some attention, and make it happen. The benefits are two-fold. That person will be uplifted and so will you because of what your act of kindness did. Doing for others, and the joy we receive from it, is medicine for our own circumstances.

So, trust God and go do good.

I said in Chapter One, my lack of trust and inability to surrender were my main missing puzzle pieces. Looking back on this experience in my life, I *know* it was that because I had tried everything else. I *know* it because I couldn't have peace without doing this act of surrender. That lack of peace kept me in a state of constant inner conflict and out of alignment, which I know now was preventing pregnancy. And the secret ingredient, the magic sauce to a breakthrough with infertility, the *ultimate missing piece* is to be aligned body, mind, and spirit. Whatever steps it takes for *that* to happen, for your body to be in congruence so it can be brought back to wholeness and primed for fertile ground, must be done. For me, it was surrender. For you, it may be something else. Surrender falls under the spirit piece of alignment for the most part, although it has elements of body and mind as well. We will be addressing body and mind in upcoming chapters, so stay tuned if you are sensing your missing piece may fall into these categories.

Looking back, I see now that I should have sought God first, *through surrender,* and let Him lead my action steps instead of going off with all guns blazing to deal with my circumstance. We even get others' opinions/advice on what we should do before we ever go to God when they aren't even sure what do with their own problems. Then, when we are desperate, and in a worse state than we were originally, we go to Him and want Him to fix our mess.

Thankfully, I'm getting better with this. Do yourself a favor and seek God first.

Remember our scale......

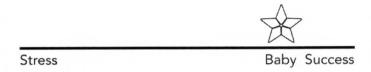

| Stress | Baby Success |

If you choose to surrender, where does that move your star? Closer to baby success or stress? If you answered baby success, you are right. Obviously, the opposite is true. Not surrendering will likely keep you in a suffering state trying to control something you can't. Let's get that star moving to the right.

The next time someone asks you what your plan is, what you are doing about your infertility, just say one thing. Say, "I'm trusting God."

Reflection and Journal Prompts

Are you in acceptance or surrender? Or neither? How can you tell?

What is your way of "being" through this? How much emotional pain are you in?

How do you manage it?

What do you need to be completely honest with yourself about?

What would freedom look like/feel like to you?

What is your worst-case scenario? What are your fears?

What is your infertility trying to teach you about yourself? About life?

What advice would *you* give to someone in your situation? Do *that*.

What is your level of trust in God? How do you know? What behaviors do you demonstrate that support your answer?

What are times in your life that you witnessed God's faithfulness? What are some examples of God coming through for you?

Trusting in God comes from experience. Draw on those times you have previously experienced trust to assist you. If you can't think of any, think about the processes of your body that happen without your conscious participation. Your heart beats, you breathe, you blink, your wounds heal, etc. That is God taking care of you. You don't have to earn this or be a good enough person for this to occur. You trust that it will just happen. Start with that.

Create a surrender prayer that comes from your heart. Declare it with conviction.

Here is a sample one.

> Jesus, I surrender myself to you.
>
> Take care of everything.
>
> I have faith the highest and best outcomes
>
> are unfolding in my life.

Chapter Four
Story

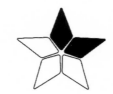

Change your story. Change your life.

—Tony Robbins

The power of our mind and the thoughts we choose to think affect our lives dramatically. Emotions are generated by these thoughts. What you think about determines how you feel. Obviously, if we change our thoughts, we can experience different emotions.

The stronger the intensity level of an emotion associated with a particular thought, the more that thought will *stick* in our brain. Your strongest memories, whether desirable or undesirable, are memorable because an intense emotion is attached to them.

Your self-talk about the events you experience reveals the meaning and perspective you give to what is happening. This is *your* story. Your story is the lens through which you view what is happening or not happening in your life. It's your take on it. It's the meaning *you* assign to it. The story we tell ourselves determines our journey and how we experience our life. Someone else may have the same event happening but have a completely different story that they tell. This *story* is point two of the Five-Point SuperStar System.

How you choose to think about your infertility will affect how you experience it and feel about it, which can influence the outcome. We often tend to focus on the fear of what we *don't* want rather than the joy of what we *do* want. For instance, with infertility, our mind can focus intently on the fear of never becoming a mother, which puts our bodies into stress mode, as opposed to purposely thinking thoughts that will provide some peace of mind. We can *choose* our thoughts. It is so important to be careful, selective, and wise about what you think about because that is what gets the ball rolling in one direction or another, and it can make all the difference.

Do you know what your thoughts are? Have you paid attention to them? It's important that you do because what we focus on (give our attention to) grows and magnifies and becomes more and more present in our life. The problem is that a lot of times we aren't aware, and these unconscious thoughts can do their dirty work without us even realizing it! We have habits of thinking a certain way and they are on autopilot. Becoming conscious of them and choosing thoughts from that awareness space is where power resides.

We have an area of our brain located in the brain stem that is called the reticular activating system (RAS), known as the "matchmaker" which creates a filter for what you give your attention to. The RAS has a job to not overload your brain with too much information. It's a gatekeeper standing guard on which sensory information you perceive from the outside world will get into your conscious mind. The RAS sorts through the information based on its relevancy to you. It only allows in what is important and of interest to you. The RAS is why after you purchase your new car, you start seeing that same make/model everywhere. Your outside world reflects back your inner thoughts like a boomerang.

The RAS will also find information that validates your beliefs in that same manner. One part of your brain *thinks* something, and another part of your brain goes on a mission to *prove* the thinker part right. The key is getting the prover to match up evidence in your life that you want and is desirable to you. How do you do that? Think the thoughts that you want to see evidence of in your life. If you think to yourself or say aloud, *I'm never going to get pregnant*, you need to start asking yourself, *Is this the story I want to match?* The belief becomes stronger the more we think it and say it.

What you think about you bring about.

Our thoughts are extremely powerful, and the beauty is that *this* is one of those areas you *do* have control of in your life. If you can gain control of your mind, your life will improve in ways you could never imagine! We want our thoughts to work for us, not against us. So, let's do this!!

This chapter will require some work from you—some inner work. I can assure you that the results from doing this will be very worth it to you. You will get out of it what you put into it. Do this for you.

Your Infertility Story

I want you to get a sense of your story around infertility. We are going to do some activities that will help bring awareness to your thoughts and beliefs.

For the first one, grab your journal and write the word *Infertility* at the top of one page. Next, I'd like you to brainstorm and brain dump anything that comes to your mind when you think about your infertility and the place it has in your life right now. Take three to four minutes to do this as you write down your thoughts quickly. Write as much as you can. It can be single words, phrases, full sentences, or a combination of these. Do not judge or overthink what comes to mind. Be spontaneous and jot it down quickly as soon as it pops into your head. There is no right or wrong thought. Don't hold back, just let it roll. Once you are finished, put this list aside for the moment.

After that, write the following sentences in your journal, and fill in the blanks with your thoughts after you write them. You may have multiple answers for these blanks, which is fine. Be as thorough as possible with your answers to Statement 1 and Statement 2.

1. What I fear the most with my infertility is _____ because if that happens that means _____.

2. My biggest fear about being pregnant is _____. My biggest fear about being a mother is _____.

Now, take a look at your brainstorming list. What do you notice? Can you identify some of your beliefs from what you have written? This is an important step because what we believe, we feel with certainty. Our belief is the toggle switch that regulates whether our body goes into that fight or flight response or rest and repair. And being too much in fight or flight can make our bodies go haywire. I would like you to work with this so you can have your thoughts serving your highest good and getting you in the direction of having your baby.

These thoughts (beliefs) affect how you feel, which then impacts the choices you make in your life. It all starts in the mind, so learning to gain control over it can be your superpower!

Here's my brain dump example:

Unfair.

Time is running out.

This isn't how it was supposed to be.

Why me?

Maybe we're too old.

What if it never happens?

I have to be a mom.

Adoption feels like I'd be giving up.

Am I being punished for my past?

I have to figure out a way.

Do we have any similarities in our lists?

Our thoughts can either empower us or disempower us.

They can be contracting or expansive.

Limiting or limitless.

How would you categorize your thoughts? I know my list of thoughts pretty much fall into disempowering, contracting, and limiting. They come from a place of lack. The two statements that contain "have to" in them indicate an internal sense of pressure. That pressure creates anxiety.

You may be thinking,

> *Well of course my thoughts would be like that. This isn't pleasant. Why would I have pleasant thoughts? I hate this situation.*

Believe me, I get it. No one is saying you aren't completely justified in having your negative thoughts. But it's critical to recognize that these thoughts don't serve you. They can create more distress in your body, which can further imbalance your hormones, which is not ideal for conception to occur. Certainly, you will have some of these thoughts at times and the feelings they generate are normal and understandable; however, you don't want to stay there.

Remember, I said our thoughts can be on autopilot and become a habit. My intent is for you to recognize these limiting beliefs now so you can interrupt them as they happen. Then you can change them into empowering beliefs that will bring about that which you desire instead of what you don't.

Thoughts are energy, and feelings are energy. We want energy that is aligned with conceiving a baby, and that takes consciously being aware of our thoughts. Each thought has a physical and an emotional reaction in the body. The average person has 12,000 to 60,000 thoughts per day, and of those thoughts we have each day, 80 percent tend to be negative and 95 percent of them tend to be repetitive—repeating that same story (National Science Foundation, 2005). So, it's easy to see how your thoughts can impact you for better or worse. You can change the story because you think the thoughts. It requires being intentional with them and aware of them.

Now, let's look at the first fill-in-the-blank statement. Our fears indicate our beliefs, and when we dig deeper and dissect them, we discover more. I'll use my own answers to model how you can work through this for yourself.

1. What I fear the most with my infertility is <u>that I may never have my own baby,</u> because if that happens that means <u>I won't be happy/fulfilled.</u>

My belief: *I can't be happy in my life unless I have a baby.*

This is a very limiting belief. It's disempowering and it's contracting. It closes me off to life. So, let's challenge this belief. Let's disprove it because it's not absolute truth.

Thought process to shift the limiting belief: I don't have a baby now. I haven't had a baby all my life, so does that mean I was never happy? Of course not. I can identify many times in my life when I was happy.

This belief needs to be changed to one that is true and is empowering, one that makes sense and that I can buy into.

New belief: *I will be able to feel happiness in my life even if I don't have my own baby because I have been happy before without one.*

That's believable, expansive, and it creates emotions that feel better than the original limiting belief.

I also filled in Statement 1's blanks with some other thoughts.

1. What I fear the most with my infertility is <u>not ever being a mother</u>, because if that happens it means <u>I would be incomplete.</u>

If we dig deeper, we ask, *Why would you feel incomplete?* My answer would be because I have always seen myself as a mother and to not be one would make me question who I really am, my purpose, my worth, and my value.

Because I had always envisioned myself as a mother and was validated in this by my love for and knack with babies and children over many years of my life, my value and worth were measured by this. Thus, creating the thought and limiting belief that follows.

My belief: *I'm not enough if I'm not a mother.*

Well, if I think and believe this, of course it would be devastating to not become a mother. I would feel a sense of desperation to pull out all the stops to get it to happen and fall into the pit of despair each time it didn't. I was operating from fear, in my ego, so I would stay consistent with how I defined myself. It was a powerful force protecting my identity. Our beliefs are potent. Even though this belief was sabotaging me, I defended it strongly in my mind to uphold my self-identity.

Remember, fear puts us out of alignment. What emotions do you think that belief created? There was fear, sadness, grief, hopelessness, and anxiety.

Medical professionals assert that a person healthy in body, mind, and spirit is considered fertile. Is capable of conceiving. The belief I had wasn't healthy by any standard.

Let's challenge this belief. Disprove it.

Thought process to shift the limiting belief: I am a wife, a sister, a daughter, an aunt, a friend, a counselor. All of these have value and worth and serve great purpose in this life, plus the fact that my worth is inherent from the start due to being created and merely being in existence on this earth. This is truth.

New belief: *Even if I am not a mother, I still matter to many people in my life.*

That is empowering. What emotions would this belief create?

Can you see and feel the power and weight our thoughts have? They can take us down a completely different road. I hope my personal examples will serve as a guide for you to rewire your own beliefs. Keep asking yourself *why* questions to get to the root so you can change your limiting belief from its core place.

Now let's look at your answers to the second set of fill-in-the blank questions. Statement 1 had you distill what your fear of infertility is, and Statement 2 takes you on an exploratory process in the opposite direction. Statement 2 leads you to identify what you may be afraid of if you would become pregnant and what fears you may have about being a mother. As odd as this may seem, there may be subconscious beliefs that were formed long ago that you have carried with you for years and are embedded. Working through these fears in the same way we did with Statement 1 will allow you to shift your story.

2. My biggest fear about being pregnant is <u>the pain of giving birth</u>. My biggest fear about being a mother is <u>that it will be difficult, and I will fail</u>.

Let's work through the example for Statement 2 together.

My Belief: *I can't deal with the pain of childbirth especially after hearing horrendous labor and delivery stories others have experienced.*

Thought Process for the Limiting Belief: It's completely normal to be nervous about something I have never experienced before. There are options available to me to manage labor pain and anxiety that I can put in place. I have dealt with pain before in my life and this pain will have a certain end to it that results in a wonderful reward.

New Belief: *I am strong and I am capable of doing hard things especially when the result is being a mother and holding my sweet baby in my arms.*

Perhaps you have other fears about giving birth, or you had a dream when you were a child that you died in childbirth. Maybe your mother wasn't in the picture while you were growing up or she was emotionally unavailable. This leaves you with strong doubts as to whether you can step up to the plate mothering a child of your own since you didn't have a strong role model for what constitutes a good mother. There are many different scenarios that could come up as answers to those questions. You may find that your fears in this area aren't even rational and that's okay. Sometimes we believe things that don't make sense but if they feel real to us, they hold power. Uncover these beliefs, disprove them because they aren't true, and substitute them with new empowering ones that *are* true just like you did with Statement 1.

Perspective Is Power

The story you spin about the events happening in your life and how you feel about them is up to you. Here's something I really want you to *get* because it will positively impact your life greatly if you do. It isn't the thing (event/circumstance) in life, whether the *thing* is being laid off from your job, a divorce, or your car breaks down, it's the meaning we give to that thing/situation. How we view it affects how we feel about it. Then, we keep thinking about it, talking about it, and beating ourselves up about it, putting that RAS to work even more.

The event in and of itself is neutral. It just is. It's a fact.

Let's take the job example. Your boss had to let three people go, and you are one of them. Bob and Sally are the other two. You and Bob commiserate about how unfair it is that you three were the unlucky ones so you bad mouth the boss and the company. You talk on the phone and rehash things you never liked about your boss and lament over how the change in finances is now going to set you back. All this negativity has you feeling depressed, tired, and now you have succumbed to eating away these feelings with your favorite ice cream each night, making you feel even worse about yourself and your current place in life. To top it off, feeling this way shortens your fuse and your tolerance level, and you find yourself snapping at your spouse and being critical of him, resulting in him starting to withdraw from you. Now, you and your hubby are either arguing or not talking at all. You want to *blame* your boss for all of this.

Sally experienced this same event. She didn't initially like this unexpected and unpreferred new direction her life had to take just like you and Bob. However, she chose to view it as an opportunity to search for a job that was an even better fit for her, one that allowed for her to grow within the company and offered her a salary that matched her skills and experience. She envisioned how this new position and salary would make her feel. She was excited that this layoff forced her to take this step because without this push she may not have taken her own initiative since it's easier to stay where you are comfortable. Her upbeat outlook motivated her to revise her résumé, start honing her interviewing skills, and begin job hunting! Sally wants to *thank* her boss for this.

Same event, different meaning. Who chooses the meaning?

You do!

When you choose the meaning, it affects your attitude.

Your attitude affects the choices you will make.

Your choices affect your outcome.

In that example, you chose to put your focus (attention) on all the things you didn't like, your boss, the company, past incidents, income reduction, and how you were the unlucky victim.

Sally chose to focus on the opportunity for the positive change this could bring in her life, imagining how she would feel when this good comes to her, and therefore, it inspired positive action.

Your story will keep you stuck, miserable, and possibly in a continual downward spiral with the negative ripple effects taking on their own momentum, unless and until you change your story. Remember what we focus on magnifies. Our outer world mirrors our internal world. They match up. Change your internal world and you change your reality.

Just look at the power of your thoughts. It's incredible how they shape your life and influence your outcomes in dramatic ways. And *you* have control over them.

So, let your thoughts work *for* you!

My husband, Tom, is very good at this. No matter what the circumstance, he remains emotionally regulated and stable. I have asked him, "How do you not get worked up over this or stressed out?" He tells me there is no point. He says his mind just starts working on the best way to solve the situation and make it better rather than dwelling on the injustice of it or how undesirable it is. He accepts *what is* and focuses on what he has control over. He doesn't make the situation worse than it is or go down the rabbit hole of worry. He stays present, practical, and solution focused. I truly believe that at seventy-one years old, his ability to have command over his mind is one of the key reasons for the optimal health he has always experienced.

The Power of Language

Let's take a look at how we can shift our perspective about infertility so that it can serve us well. We already know the disempowering thoughts and meanings we can give it. We are all good at that. Just refer to the brain dump you did earlier as proof.

Let's view infertility another way—an empowering way.

First off, I say we get rid of the word *infertility*. Ugh. I detest that word. Language and word choice is huge when it comes to mindset and how a particular word can evoke a certain emotion.

The World Health Organization defines infertility as the *inability/failure* to become pregnant after one year or more of regular unprotected sexual intercourse. It can be primary in which a pregnancy has never occurred or secondary where one or both members of the couple have previously conceived but are unable to again after a full year of trying. Dictionary.com defines *infertility* as the *persistent inability* to achieve conception and produce an offspring.

Infertility is linked to the word *inability*, which is synonymous with *unable*, *incapable*, *failure,* and *ineptitude*. How do these words make you feel?

Empowered? Inspired? Hopeful? Confident?

Absolutely not. Probably the complete opposite.

I say we change the word to something that is truth because that is key. It needs to be believable and allow us to feel hopeful and empowered. We have the choice to do that! The medical community may not adopt our new lingo (for now anyway), but for our purposes in this book and staying consistent with flipping our story, let's change it.

Let's think this through.

I have an issue with the word *inability* being used to define infertility. Inability means not able, so following suit, infertility means not fertile. The diagnostic term of infertility is fundamentally negative and is both contracting and limiting. Not good for the mindset whatsoever.

You may not be fertile at this very moment, but it doesn't mean you won't ever be or that you aren't capable of being fertile, barring any major anatomical reasons that would make it impossible to conceive and bear a child (like having no uterus or something of that nature). You may be experiencing secondary infertility, so that alone indicates that the possibility is there. You may have undetermined infertility, which although not having any specific findings for your fertility issues is extremely frustrating, it also means it's very possible, and it just hasn't happened yet. This doesn't equate to unable or inability.

If our body, mind, and spirit are healthy, fertility is possible. Something is out of sync, out of balance, and getting in the way of that alignment, which is what this book is helping you to uncover for yourself. If we bring ourselves back to the wholeness state, we *are* then free to conceive. You aren't conceiving because conditions aren't ideal for it to occur at this point, not that you are always going to be unable to.

In essence, until that alignment happens and stays stable, your fertility is on hold, delayed, postponed, suspended, challenged, or interrupted. That sounds temporary, right? It is unlike the word *infertility* with its inability connotation which sounds permanent and fixed.

Take a look at these alternative word choices and their meanings.

Delayed—occurring more slowly than normal, expected, or desired; or to stop for a time (that's true).

Suspended—Merriam-Webster states that *suspend* implies temporary stoppage with an added suggestion of waiting until some condition is satisfied (that's also true).

Challenged—Cambridge English Dictionary defines it as having a physical or mental condition that makes ordinary activities more difficult than they are for other people (hmmm…that's certainly true).

Which word empowers you more? Perhaps you have come up with one I didn't list. I personally tend to lean more toward the word *challenged* because I like a challenge, so I relate positively to this word.

Let's try it on. Say these statements to yourself and out loud and see how they make you feel. What emotions do they evoke within you?

I am infertile.

I am fertility challenged.

When I say these two statements, the first one makes me feel like it's a lost cause, a done deal. The second statement makes me feel like I'm not where I want to be and it may be a bit of a struggle to get there, but that there is hope and possibility. There's still an open door. It feels so much lighter.

How do these two statements feel to you? Do you notice any difference between the two? You may prefer the words *delayed* or *suspended* more.

Just this small shift in thinking can make you feel differently and as a result behave differently. Your body responds differently to the feeling as well.

This one small change of wording is a completely different story that you tell yourself.

If we go back to that Dictionary.com definition and replace the word *inability* with *challenge*, it would read as this: The persistent *challenge* to achieve conception and produce an offspring. Sounds like a better definition, one that is achievable, providing that glimmer of hope. Heck, you have overcome challenges in your life before.

Because our thoughts are so powerful, I think it would be wise to use the term *fertility challenged* in place of infertility for the remainder of this book. The more you see it, say it, believe it, and feel it, the more it becomes a new habit and can produce good fruit. I invite you to do this so you can set the stage for positive change and create the reality you desire.

I would even suggest that you take it another step and refer to yourself as an expectant mama-to-be because you *are expecting to be a mother.* That is absolute truth.

I am an expectant mama-to-be. How does that feel? Refer to yourself in this beautiful way.

The words *I am* hold an incredible amount of power, so be very selective of what you put behind them. Forget your limiting diagnosis and all the yuck that comes with it. *Stop* saying you have that diagnosis. *Stop* saying it to yourself, to your spouse, to your friends, to your family, to your coworkers. *Stop* saying it period. Start saying regularly with a smile on your face and in your heart, and with complete trust, *I am an expectant mama-to-be* and let the RAS do its job for you. Let the prover prove your thinker right!

How else can you shift your view of being fertility challenged? This diagnosis doesn't have to be some cruel curse that's been imposed on you shattering your dreams and happiness. You *can choose* to view it as your messenger telling you that your body is out of balance, and it is feedback for you to get curious and do some investigating about what needs to change to get back on track and in alignment. Incidentally, this book is your partner in this investigation.

The knowledge you acquire from doing this and putting that knowledge into practice in your life can be transformative and prevent similar situations down the road. Being fertility challenged is a wake-up call. It's your chance to do things differently to improve your life in all aspects that may never have happened otherwise. Your thinking got you where you are and now it's time for next level thinking for your next level of life. You can't get something new and different (your baby) doing what you've always done. One day you may even see it as a gift.

Seek and You Shall Find

The really amazing thing about a cloudy day is that the sun is still shining. It is still there. It's just covered by the clouds. There *is* light through the darkness and heaviness of being fertility challenged. Where will you put your focus? On the clouds? Or on the light that you know is there? What we put our attention on, we find more of.

You must look for the light (be willing and open to changing thoughts, beliefs, perspectives, and choices that don't serve you well).

- Look for the light in being completely honest with yourself.

- Look for the light in the lessons to be learned and the opportunity for it.

- Look for the light in discovering yourself through this process.

- Look for the light because it's the way out of the darkness.

- Look for the light in your faith that God is comforting you and walking beside you the whole time. Look for His signs of this. They are there.

- Look for the light in your new story. It has the power to change your life.

- Look for the light in your recognition that you hold the power within you to create your desired reality.

- Look for the light in what resonates with you throughout this book. This light is your way through this.

- Follow the light, believe in the light, and let it guide you. Do the exercises and reflections in this book, take positive action, create new patterns and habits, and experience your breakthrough as the light completely breaks through your clouds, mama.

Reflections and Journal Prompts

Explore your beliefs on motherhood. Do a brain dump on this topic.

Why do you want to be a mother?

What do you think defines a good mother?

Are there expectations regarding a timeline for it to occur? (i.e., before you turn a certain age.)

Whose expectations are they?

What is your story about how motherhood *has* to look? What are your rules around it? Will you *only* consider having a child that is biologically yours? Are you open to other avenues such as egg donor, sperm donor, surrogacy, adoption, embryo adoption, or fostering?

Consider why or why not? Our values and needs get intertwined with our beliefs.

Sift out whether the values are really yours or if they are someone else's.

This is a big area of contemplation and worth digging into, particularly if you and your spouse have different opinions about how you are willing to become parents or if you have never broached the topic.

Keep in mind that *fixed* mindsets create more emotional pain. Do you have a fixed mindset on what motherhood *has* to look like? If motherhood for you can *only* be bearing your own biological child, explore why that is the case. What are you making it mean about you if it doesn't happen that way? What are you making it mean about you if you would choose another option? These are important things to understand about yourself.

Sorting through this will help you determine if you value being a mother in general *more* than requiring it to be a child you conceive and give birth to. One way is more expansive, and the other is limiting. This is your journey. You get to decide. Do yourself the favor of identifying your beliefs in this area and rewiring them as we have done before if you feel inclined to do that.

What are your beliefs about your body? What is the story you tell yourself about your body these days? Do you need a *new* story that puts you in the driver's seat on your road to motherhood?

As a quick wrap-up, where does a story of limiting beliefs move your *star* on our scale?

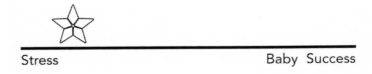

Stress   Baby Success

(Answer: Limiting beliefs move you to the left toward stress and away from your goal. I'm positive you got the answer correct!)

Where will your new story put your *star*?

What is your *new* story? Write it down and read it before going to sleep.

With all that you have learned about yourself in this chapter, would you identify your *story* as one of your main missing pieces to attaining your heart's desire?

Chapter Five

State

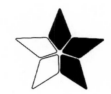

There is a unique pain that comes from
preparing a place in your heart for a child that
never comes.

—David Platt

Tony Robbins, author and world-renowned transformational
speaker, always says in his Unleash the Power Within trainings that
the quality of our life is where we live emotionally. That means that
the level of satisfaction we experience in our life is relative to what
our dominant emotional state is. Think about where *you* are living
emotionally right now. How about the past six months? The past
year or two? What has been your dominant emotion throughout the
day? Certainly, our feelings may fluctuate throughout the day at
times, but we have an emotional set point that we settle into
naturally. That emotional state is point three of the Five-Point
SuperStar System.

Being fertility challenged is all-encompassing. It affects you physically, mentally, emotionally, and spiritually. It can feel like it's taking over who you are with the biological desperation to make getting pregnant happen. Living with this day to day, month to month, year to year, can put you in a state of anger, frustration, disappointment, anxiety, depression, and even hopelessness. Remember, as we have discussed, our external world mirrors our internal world. That internal emotional state could mirror things showing up in your life that bring on more frustration, disappointment, sadness, and anger. The good news is that we can *choose* to live emotionally in a joyful state so we can enjoy our lives a lot more and bring even more of that abundance into them.

Just like we have belief/thought patterns, we can also have patterns of emotion. We think that's who we are. I *am* depressed. I *am* a worry wart. We *aren't* our feelings. We are *feeling* these feelings, but we *aren't* those feelings. We are separate from them. The more we identify ourselves *as* them, that is what we see in our lives and attract more of. We live up to that identity like a self-fulfilling prophecy. Remember, we talked about being careful about what you put after the words *I am*. It is powerful. I *am* strong. I *am* hopeful. I *am* loving. I *am* capable of all things. I *am* whole. Now, we're talking!

What is your relationship with your feelings? Do you express them in a healthy way and in a timely manner? Or do you stuff them, avoid them, or deny them? Do you distract yourself from feeling them and numb yourself to them by engaging in behaviors like social media, shopping, drinking, food indulgence, drinking alcohol, overworking, or TV watching? What is your pattern? Be honest with yourself.

As you read on, see if you relate in any way to what I am sharing. For many, many years of my life I was a people pleaser. Making and keeping other people in my life happy was how I learned to receive the basic need of love and connection. I would often compromise my own needs, wants, thoughts, and desires in order to earn approval, acknowledgment, and love from those I believed were important to please. This became a conditioned response when I was a little girl and remained so well into my forties, until I did a lot of self-development and grew in this area.

In my first marriage, the counselor I was seeing labeled me codependent because I prioritized the needs of my husband and significant others in my life over my own. My thinking and behavior centered around them and their needs so they could be happy. If they were happy, then I felt love and connection, and I could be happy. So, basically, my feelings weren't really my own. They were *dependent* on others' feelings. I was disconnected from them. I didn't really know what I felt because I always pushed my feelings aside and took on what I believed would be approved of and have me be seen in a positive light. My relationship with my feelings wasn't a good one and I paid a price for it. Hopefully, what we cover in this chapter will encourage you to foster a healthy relationship with your feelings.

Unfortunately, many of us as children were discouraged from expressing our feelings. We were told, "Stop crying before I give you something to cry about" or "Smile" or "Don't be such a baby" or "You're fine" or "Be a big girl." We interpreted this to mean that our feelings (and sometimes even ourselves) were not acceptable, appropriate, or okay, or didn't matter. Our protective ego and defense mechanisms resorted to suppressing, ignoring, and not acknowledging these feelings. Essentially, we shut down and tucked those feelings away. But they needed to go somewhere. They didn't just disappear. Over time, this emotional energy builds up and forms blockages in the body and can have physical manifestations if it isn't released. Emotional blockages can become physical blockages.

People are uncomfortable with unpreferred feelings like sadness, anger, or frustration. This discomfort motivates us to get those feelings to be over with quickly, to deny them, or to redirect them. Feelings aren't *good* or *bad.* They just *are.* They are part of our human experience. This is why I use the words *preferred* or *unpreferred* instead of good or bad. We ended up concluding that certain feelings were bad because we felt the need to shut them down for parent approval.

Feelings are very helpful. They provide us feedback. The preferred ones like happiness, joy, peace, love, free, and content indicate to us to keep doing what we are doing to keep experiencing them. We are on the right track. The unpreferred ones like anger, jealousy, resentment, loneliness, or sadness tell us that something needs to be changed, dealt with, or adjusted. They are messengers to get our attention and show us that we aren't dealing with something and it's putting us out of alignment.

The unpreferred ones may not feel pleasant, but they also allow us to really appreciate the preferred ones. We need this contrast for direction. We wouldn't know joy without sadness and so forth. As human beings, we are meant to experience the full spectrum of feelings.

Habits Are Hard to Break

Even with my own fertility challenges, I found myself in the same pattern of sending my emotions away. I put on a stiff upper lip every day at work as an elementary school counselor despite having to work alongside pregnant colleagues. I gave my whole heart to the precious children I served, which only intensified my desire to have my own children to raise and cherish.

I didn't really open up to my husband about how distraught I truly was that we couldn't conceive. Sure, he knew how important it was to me, but the deep level of grief I had about it I held tightly. I guess I didn't want him to give up our wide range of efforts we were trying in order to conceive if he knew it was upsetting me to that degree. I also didn't want him to take any of it on personally and have it potentially negatively impact his performance in the bedroom. So, most of our discussions about it typically centered around the logistics of whatever strategy we were implementing at the time and not discussing or processing our emotions about it all.

At work and at home, I didn't want to burden others with my intense emotions and, if I'm being honest, I didn't want to appear out of control. I wanted to maintain my stoicism and my independence of being able to handle everything on my own. I pretended it was a strength not to express my feelings, when in fact, it takes great courage and strength to be vulnerable and share emotions. I was hiding from mine. Where is the strength in pretending and hiding? I was fooling myself.

I have a feeling that many of us struggling with fertility challenges share a similar personality profile. We are fiercely independent, like to be in control, are determined, go-getters, givers to our own detriment, and we measure our self-worth by it. When it comes to our feelings, we need to loosen that control. A lot.

Feelings that don't get healthy expression can come out in physical manifestations as in physical ailments like headaches or backaches or anxiety or depression. If it's over a long period of time, it can physically manifest as disease. For so many years, I suppressed my feelings, and they manifested in high levels of anxiety, IBS, depressive episodes, and hormonal imbalances. This is why I mentioned earlier in the stress chapter that it's possible we may have unintentionally brought on the fertility challenges we are experiencing. Habitual patterns of trying to control our emotions and poor coping skills to manage our stress don't serve us well.

Given the level of distress that fertility challenges can cause, not expressing/processing feelings in healthy ways will continue to keep you out of alignment, making conception less likely to occur. We certainly don't want that. We don't want to continue ways that haven't been working for us. So, we are going to discuss what processing your feelings in healthy ways looks like. We are also going to address two BIG emotional patterns that, if left unattended, can really keep you stuck, blocked energetically, and out of alignment.

The simplest and most straight forward advice I can give you when it comes to expressing your feelings in a healthy way is to feel your feelings organically in the way that a baby does.

What does that mean?

Babies don't judge themselves for *having* feelings, and they don't judge the *feeling* they are experiencing.

Babies don't resist their feelings, they let them *be*; they allow them.

Babies don't attach any meaning to their feelings, not good or bad, not right or wrong, they just are.

Now, let me give you a little bit more than that since you are way more sophisticated than a baby. When you feel painful emotions, express them as they come up. Feel them and release them.

Sit with the feeling. Notice the sensation in your body, the energy of it. Where do you feel it? Is it in your head, throat, jaw, chest, or stomach? Or somewhere else? Does it feel hot, warm, or cold? Tense, heavy, or light? Observe it. Become aware of thoughts you may be having that can help you identify the feeling. Do you feel a nudge to repress it or move away from the feeling? Why? Continue to stay with it.

Sometimes we think the feeling will be too much for us and overwhelm us or we think it will never end. Perhaps the way this is presented is new to you. Take some time getting used to it as it may be a new way of dealing with feelings, and it may be uncomfortable. That's okay; it will end, and you will be better for it. Breathing through it will help. Breathe in for the count of five, hold for the count of five, and then exhale for the count of five. Do it several times.

Consider the following as you sit with the feeling:

What time frame is this upset in? Is it about something in the past or the future?

Is there a need that isn't being met? (Do you feel like you are not being heard, or are you lacking the feeling of belonging, respect, safety, attention, relief, certainty, control, or peace of mind?)

How else can you meet that need without feeling this stress?

What can you uncover about what the feeling is trying to give you feedback on so you can better understand it? Christine Breese, a speaker at a parenting summit I attended, suggests asking yourself the following questions when emotions come up for you:

What am I not noticing that I need to pay attention to?

Are there some limits to set, lines to be drawn, or boundaries I need to put in place or enforce?

Does something in my environment need to be different?

Is there a relationship that isn't healthy for me that I need to recognize?

Is there something I need to do or change?

What is preventing me in this moment from experiencing joy?

Journaling is a great way to process your feelings. Seeing your thoughts on paper (and out of your head) about what you are feeling helps you to make sense of them. The act of writing helps you to confront your feelings instead of hiding from them. Once you identify the message from the feeling and address it with actions that are congruent with that newfound clarity, the feeling will go on its merry way. Even if you are not a writer this can be an effective way to work through emotions. Don't "write it off" before trying it!

Talking through feelings with a trusted friend or family member, life coach, or therapist is another way to release and process them in a healthy way.

Exercising, dancing, massage, yoga, creative outlets, and self-care practices are other healthy examples of emotional release.

The goal isn't to *control* your emotions, to tough it out, or just get over it. You need to *feel* your feelings. That's why the root word in feelings is *feel*. We need to move *through them,* so they move through our body and don't get stuck. Remember our discussion on surrender and the value of it? Do this with your feelings as well. Surrender to your feelings. Allow them, acknowledge them, and be open. Don't resist them. What we resist persists. Noticing, acknowledging, validating, expressing, and processing our feelings is the best way to heighten our dominant emotional state long term. It can take some time to get to those emotions that we have been so good at denying by pretending everything is fine, so be patient and compassionate with yourself.

Dealing with Grief

Many years ago, I attended a professional conference on grief and loss and the speaker posed this question to us:

> Which type of death causes more grief? An anticipated death of a loved one as with a terminal illness or a sudden/unexpected death of a loved one as with an accident or crime?

What would your answer be?

The answer is that they are both heavily grief ridden but in different ways. One isn't necessarily worse than the other. The sudden death brings on acute grief with the shock component because there was no mental preparation for it, no time to get things in order, and no opportunity for a goodbye. Often, there can be survivor's guilt attached and the aftermath of investigations and legal proceedings that continue for years bringing on additional stress.

The anticipated death grief process entails hearing/accepting the diagnosis of the loved one and your support of them in a multitude of ways throughout the experience while also coping with your own emotions that arise from it all. The grief is constant as each day exposes you to new situations surrounding the illness as you wonder if this is your last day, your last moment with your loved one. You face the grief daily.

In both these situations, grief is being experienced from the loss of what *used to be.*

I bring this distinction to your attention with an intent to get you to recognize the *validity* and the *depth* of grief that can accompany fertility challenges. The grief is real, and it needs to be recognized and expressed by you.

In *your* situation, you are experiencing grief from the loss of what *has never been,* loss from a broken dream, and of a highly valued stage of life of an expected family. Childlessness is a significant trauma for a woman who desperately wants to be a mother.

Not only is the grief from fertility challenges profound, but also the losses are intensified by their lack of visibility and the lack of understanding by society. This makes the sufferer feel more isolated in their grief and less supported.

I want to make you aware of the magnitude of grief that can be experienced with fertility challenges so that you don't inadvertently minimize it or suppress it because you feel like no one really understands what you're going through, making you question whether you have a right to this grief at all. This grief is real; it is valid and profound, despite whether others understand it or acknowledge it. It is essential that you affirm this and give yourself permission to feel it and move through it.

Let me illustrate the layers of loss that compound with the following diagram. The diagram of sand in a bottle simulates how each unique loss (layer of sand) creates a compound effect of grief.

Layers of Loss

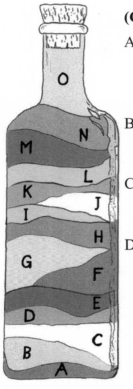

(Compounded Grief)

A. Initial grief response when pregnancy isn't occurring; not being able to do what is expected after trying to conceive for a significant period of time.

B. Receiving the diagnosis for your fertility issues, or despite comprehensive testing it remains undetermined.

C. The arrival of each monthly cycle reminds you of how far away you are from what you desire most.

D. Engaging in medical interventions like the complex process of ART is emotionally draining with the required hormone shots further intensifying emotions. Failed medical interventions are a roller coaster with high hopes felt for them to work and loss of hope when they don't. And if you choose not to pursue these at all, there is coping with the ramifications of that.

E. The meaning that is attached to these losses further compounds the pain such as missing out on:

*a positive pregnancy test and the excitement/planning of sharing that news with your spouse, family/friends.

*first ultrasound visit and coveted picture from it.

*hearing baby's heartbeat.

*experiencing the miracle of carrying a baby that grows inside your womb.

*capturing the beauty and memory with pregnancy photos and belly molds.

*the celebratory baby shower.

*genetic legacy (surname).

*passing on traditions.

*planning for or imagining grandparenthood.

These repeated losses are felt with each monthly cycle that arrives, with each failed medical intervention, and with each reminder mentioned in the next layer (F).

F. Being surrounded by reminders regularly like friends and family with children (attending birthday parties, school/ educational milestones, holiday celebrations, special events, sports games), baby showers, gender reveal parties, Facebook posts of new baby arrivals and children in general, and the **all-time biggie**, Mother's Day.

G. Silently suffering because no one really seems to get it unless they have gone through it. Others tread lightly not knowing what to say and often their comments can come off inconsiderate and insensitive like "Give it time" or "You can always adopt" or "Just relax" or "Maybe it's divine will and you're not meant to have children" or "Have you tried _____?" The implications of these comments can make you feel inadequate or that you aren't trying hard enough. I remember when I was working in the school as an elementary school counselor and in the throes of ART I would hear a few times, "You should hang out with the teachers in the first-grade wing. They just drink the water down there and get pregnant." These comments, although not ill intended, can make you feel unseen, unheard, and not understood. Feeling that way can tend to make you withdraw more from others and exacerbate the loneliness of this condition.

H. The stigma surrounding being fertility challenged intensifies the atmosphere of silence. Women are socialized at a young age to train themselves for motherhood down the road through childhood play of house, babysitting, and sibling responsibilities. Although choosing not to have children is becoming more acceptable, the expectation of motherhood is still quite prevalent. This, along with the fact that the topic is infrequently discussed publicly, brings on feelings of shame or failure, which is perpetuated by society.

I. There is typically a lack of support with being fertility challenged stemming from the hidden nature of it. In a traditional and widely understood loss, like death, the griever's loss is easily identified and understood by others. Support is shown by condolences given, expressions of sympathy in the form of words, cards, flowers, cooked meals, visits, and attending the funeral or wake which helps to facilitate the grief process for the griever. Time off from work for bereavement may be given and there are fond memories to reflect on. This grief is acknowledged, validated, and supported in a variety of ways. The grief process with fertility challenges isn't linear like that. The losses are *continual*, which makes them unique. The grief is *active* and doesn't have a sense of closure.

J. There is often an internal struggle with self-loathing, self-blame, and self-judgment. (One might question if she is being punished for life decisions in the past.)

K. Dealing with disappointing your family members who are chomping at the bit to become grandparents or being judged for the unnatural methods you choose to use to become a mother and start a family may begin to affect daily life.

L. The struggling with self-identity becomes a part of who you are. It's the natural role of a woman to be able to conceive and bear children. There can be significant pain from feeling abnormal, inadequate, and not enough, as well as anger toward your body for failing you.

M. Pregnancy loss may happen over and over, thereby replaying some of the earlier pains as many women have multiple miscarriages.

N. Many experience an expedited loss of youth. The time pressure imposed due to age or the specifics of the diagnosis, as well as the prolonged nature of the condition, has menopause looming in the backdrop.

O. The decision to remain childless, to adopt, to foster, or to become a parent in an alternative way results in the loss of ever bearing your own natural child, thereby resulting in the loss of the dream.

As you can see from this extensive list, the number of losses is many, and they are profound. When coupled with not feeling seen, heard, and understood, which are fundamental human needs, the deep pain compounds. It can be a lonely place. You may have been mourning the losses of this desired life stage but not able to really articulate them. Hopefully, this diagram enables you to identify more clearly where all this emotional pain is coming from.

Mamas-to-be, it is so essential that you recognize the importance of grieving these losses as well as the uniqueness of each of them. Because this loss process is active, constant, and prolonged by its nature, there isn't a distinct endpoint to it, as with a death, where healing can officially begin. It doesn't follow the same path.

Give yourself permission to feel this grief, this sorrow. It's not about wallowing in it or taking on a victim role, but rather cleansing your heart and mind by allowing your body to feel the sensation of it. Because there are so many layers of loss, you will more than likely experience it in waves, pockets of strong emotion, and then pockets of space. The only way out of it is through it however you need to do it—scream, cry, talk with a professional, journal, exercise, massage/bodywork, dance, or yoga.

My Grief Release Freed Me

I clearly remember the day I finally dealt with my grief and experienced the cathartic relief of all I had been holding on to. Kathleen, one of my best friends, came to my house for a visit. We chatted about many topics and of course got into how I was doing emotionally with my situation. I remember for the first time *fully* letting go and eventually wailing uncontrollably in her arms as she embraced me in a comforting hug until I was done. There were loud sobbing noises, and my body was trembling as my compassionate friend was completely present with me and just allowed this release to take its course. I am so happy that I allowed myself to let loose and not continue to contain it. That emotional release, bigger than I had ever experienced before, allowed me to open my heart fully to the good that was already in my life, and it set the stage for more of it to come my way.

Sure, I had had conversations with friends and family prior to this one, and tears were shed, but there was always a piece of me that controlled my reaction, my emotional level. Some bits of grief dribbled out I'm sure, but I definitely held back. But not this time. I think I resisted feeling these emotions full out because I didn't want to fully accept the reality of my "inconceivable" situation. Not feeling that grief and avoiding it encouraged it to linger and persist. When I stepped into it fully, without keeping a check on myself and remaining in emotional control, that intense grief dissipated. Moving through it cleared it away and made space for what I was desiring to come my way. Feeling your feelings fully is *freeing*.

I do believe completely surrendering to the grief brought me clarity, a sense of peace, and is what enabled me to take the *next* transformational step in my journey to motherhood. I want that for you too.

I strongly encourage you to take a close look at where you are in the grieving process. Have you permitted yourself to fully feel your grief? Resisting it and controlling it will not help you. You must *feel* to heal.

Grieve mama-to-be. Grieve.

> Forgiveness doesn't make the other person
> right, it makes you free.
>
> —Stormie Omartian

Forgiveness is another decision you can make that can create space for receiving what you most desire and increasing your emotional set point.

We can have misconceptions about forgiveness. It can be perceived as weak or losing if you forgive the person for the pain they inflicted upon you. In fact, the opposite is true. It is the highest form of love to be able to forgive someone, particularly without them asking for it. That takes strength. Clinging to the hurt, hate, anger, resentment, and bitterness creates a barrier for divine love and peace to flow through you. Those heavy feelings eat away at you and steal your peace and joy. Forgiveness is such a *freeing* act because it opens your heart and removes the heaviness that you have been carrying around everywhere. When you heal, you open your heart, and you open up space for love, joy, and peace to fill it. That isn't losing. That's winning.

Forgiveness doesn't mean you condone what was done to you or another. It doesn't mean you approve of it, or you are excusing it, forgetting it, or justifying it. You don't forgive to release that person from what they have done. You do it to release yourself from that negative energy. You do it *for you* so you can live more fully and have peace. Leave it to God to handle their offense. It's not your burden to take on. Free yourself.

Keep in mind that holding on to those feelings of resentment, hate, and bitterness isn't payback to the person at all. They are likely going on merrily with their life completely unaware of what you are doing to yourself in your effort to "show them." It gives them power over you and keeps you bound to them emotionally. This person hurt you initially and now you are fanning the flames by hurting yourself through unforgiveness. When you forgive that person, you only have to do it once, but when you *choose not to*, you have to make that unforgiveness decision every day as you replay the pain of the event in your mind over and over, keeping it alive and giving it power over you. That's a lot of work and poor use of precious energy spent at something that doesn't serve your wellbeing at all.

Sometimes the one we need to forgive is ourselves if we are riddled with guilt, shame, or embarrassment for an action we took or something we said. Perhaps it's even a decision you made, past or present, that you think could be playing a part in your fertility challenges you have been dealt. It doesn't matter whether your conclusion is true, but if you *believe* it's true and are punishing yourself for it, then it is getting in the way. Show yourself some grace and compassion and forgive yourself. Let it go. God already has forgiven you. It's time you do the same. If you have trouble forgiving yourself, that speaks to your low level of self-worth, which we will address in the next chapter.

Going to God to answer your prayer of bestowing you with your blessing while you still have unforgiveness in your heart is probably counterproductive. God is all about forgiveness. Ask Him to reveal to you if your heart is holding on to any unforgiveness. Sometimes it has been a pattern for so long it may be unrecognizable.

Forgiveness gifts you with inner peace. Forgivers who maintain an attitude of forgiveness have realized it is the pathway to peace, love, and joy. Give yourself the gift of forgiveness and you will change your future.

The benefits of forgiveness positively impact your emotional health in that it decreases stress and anxiety levels which as a result improves your immune function and can improve your sleep. You are honoring yourself when you forgive because you are releasing yourself from the grip of this heavy load of emotions you have been tethered to and, by this, you are affirming that you do indeed deserve happiness.

So how do you forgive? Do you just say the words "I forgive you" and the pain magically goes away? It's not that easy, unfortunately. First of all, you need to have a genuine willingness to forgive. Don't do it because you will appease someone else if you do, or even because I am showing you the importance of it here and you want to check it off the list. If you forgive begrudgingly, you will have only replaced the anger/bitterness energy with reluctant/resistive energy which is not of good will and defeats the purpose.

I think a great way to forgive is to write a forgiveness letter to the person, whether that person is dead or alive, whether you still have contact with that person or not, and whether that person is *you* or even God.

In the upcoming Reflections and Journal Prompt section at the end of this chapter, I will give you a format for the letter that will guide you through the forgiveness process. If you choose to speak face to face with this person, you can use the same format to prepare your speech. You could also read your letter in person or send your letter, but neither of those is necessary for forgiveness to occur for yourself. Just writing the letter while in your heart space (centered/grounded) and never sending it will be enough for forgiveness to occur in your soul.

How do you know if you have *really* forgiven?

When your memories of the incident resurface (and they probably will), you may feel sadness rather than venomous rage about it and for the person as well. Keep the letter you wrote handy because rereading it will reinforce your commitment to forgiveness. And be ready for miracles to occur because they often come to a heart that is open and free.

Let's revisit our scale.

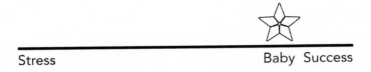

Stress   Baby Success

Which direction do you think the *star* moves when you feel your feelings and process them in a healthy way? How about when you fully grieve your losses and gift yourself with forgiveness? That's right—toward lightness, flow, and freedom—which brings you closer to your desire. Suppressing your feelings, avoiding grieving, and resisting forgiveness brings on suffering, taking you down the road of misery and stress, moving you away from the dream of your baby.

Forgiveness is the magnet which draws your endless good. It wipes clean the slate of the past to let you receive the present.

—Catherine Ponder

Reflections and Journal Prompts

What is your emotional set point?

What is your daily dominant emotion?

Track your feelings throughout the day to determine it if you are unsure. You may surprise yourself. Set your phone alarm every one or two hours for several days and document your feelings when it goes off. They don't need to be consecutive days in a row. Just several days to get an accurate picture. Assess your results at the end of each day and compare the days. This is a good exercise to do even if it's just to get you more aware of your feelings in general.

How do you handle your feelings? Do you control them or allow them? What changes do you need to make and/or what can you implement to promote a healthy expression of your feelings?

Contemplate your level of grief. Surrender to it when it arises.

Write a forgiveness letter if you have discovered there is unforgiveness in your heart and if you are willing to do so. Use the following format as a guide to structure the letter.

A. Get specific about the pain this caused you. Describe your anger and various feelings along with what it has meant to be subject to this pain.

B. Make a declaration about choosing to not allow these feelings to have power over you anymore. (*I no longer wish to feel...*)

C. This is the section where you say, "I forgive you for treating me _____." This is where you communicate that you realize that hurting people hurt people, and we are all flawed. This person was acting from their own limiting beliefs—their conditioning—and were doing the best they could with the pain and hurt they have endured in their life, likely trying to get a need met.

D. Consider *why* the person went about meeting this need in such a hurtful way. This helps you to have compassion and empathy and take it less personally. You *offer* this forgiveness just as you would hope to *receive* it, through the eyes of love in which God sees us all.

Chapter Six
Self

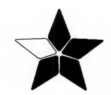

The most important relationship you have is with
yourself. Everything happening in your life
results from the way you treat yourself through
thoughts, words, and actions.

—Roxana Jones

At this point, I am certain that you realize the power of your
thoughts (beliefs, perspective, mindset, attitude) and how these
thoughts have a profound effect on how you feel and the choices
you make as a result.

I believe the thoughts we think are greatly influenced by how we
feel about ourselves—our level of self-worth. It's the undercurrent
that drives our thoughts. The power that our self-worth holds is
huge. When we believe we aren't worthy or lovable, we often seek
love outside of ourselves to fill us up and compensate for the
emptiness. This can get sticky. When we don't know our own worth

and live our lives from this place, we tend to seek others' approval, attention, and opinions to fill this unmet need for love.

I can say beyond any shadow of a doubt that one of the biggest and most meaningful favors you can do for yourself that will allow you to harness your personal power to positively influence your life so you can serve yourself and others in the greatest capacity, is to truly know your own worth. Getting a handle on this will transform you and the quality of your life! This is why *Self* is point four of the SuperStar System.

As a woman, there is a natural biological function to be able to conceive a baby. We assume the body will do this just as it performs all its other functions. It's part of our makeup and is just expected. When it doesn't, we can believe something is wrong with us—that we are greatly flawed and somehow not enough. It can understandably rattle our self-worth when conception doesn't happen.

The BIG question is how would you define your level of self-worth even prior to trying to conceive a baby? I want you to really consider this as you read on and be completely honest with yourself.

You see when your level of self-worth is low, you are more subject to the following:

- Jealousy
- Criticism
- Cynicism
- Comparing yourself to others
- Being a "doormat"/people-pleasing tendencies
- Accepting/tolerating mistreatment/disrespect
- Judgment of self/others
- Shaming of self/others
- Blaming self/others/life conditions

- Not taking personal responsibility and having a victim mentality
- Seeking validation/acceptance/approval/attention from others
- Trusting others over yourself
- Having low expectations for yourself, i.e., partner choice, job capability/salary
- Difficulty making decisions
- Concern over how you are perceived and others' opinions of you
- Identity issues
- Decreased ambition and motivation

Do you remember that my typical m.o. was to work hard at something and then I'd generally achieve it? I would set my sights on what I wanted, explore all avenues to get me there, and then make it happen. That performing to achieve was a strong pattern in my life because the positive attention/approval/validation I received from others as a result gave me a sense of worthiness and value. I learned from a very young age how getting A's, receiving positive report card comments, getting glowing remarks at parent/teacher conferences, completing my chores, having "good" behavior, and following the rules was preferred and pleasing to my parents and teachers. When they were happy, I felt love and connection. Maintaining this level of performance was a priority for me. It made me feel seen and met a basic need we all have, which is to feel significant.

My achievements took this path. I remember as early as first grade in elementary school being given the challenge of writing the numbers 1 to 1,000 on handwriting sheets and my *having* to meet that laborious challenge. I remember *having* to be the *first* one to complete the front and back of a math workbook page perfectly to get a star on it from the teacher and hear how impressed she was at how fast I could do it. I strived to win the best speller award in fifth grade which meant getting 100 percent on every spelling test the entire school year. I then topped that off in sixth grade by winning first place in the district spelling bee. I was in the accelerated program in high school and a member of the National Honor Society. I attained a BS in elementary education and then my MA in counseling psychology. I then attained certification in elementary school counseling. During those years I entered several beauty pageants (Miss USA and Miss America at local levels), swimsuit competitions, and I even pursued modeling.

I often held several jobs at a time while attending school to acquire my degrees. I continually sought out different occupations in my field that challenged me and "filled me up." I then became an entrepreneur, creating my own product for parents to use with their children, and took on the comprehensive role of managing all the spinning pieces of being a business owner. I then dabbled in something completely different for three years (direct sales) and was promoted to director in the global company within a short period of time. My latest achievement was attaining my coaching certification as a Love and Authenticity Practitioner. Always looking for the *next* thing.

My mother would often say when we would play games as a family growing up that I was a sore loser. It's become very clear to me as to why that was the case. I have always been competitive. I want to win and when I don't, I feel upset with myself.

Why?

Because as you can see, my self-worth and identity has been tied up in achieving, winning, and performing at my best. And when I don't, subconsciously my self-worth takes a hit. A person has a lot wrapped up in winning when value is defined by it.

You may read this and say that I must have had self-confidence to do well in all those endeavors and compete on stage in pageants and swimsuit competitions, so how could my self-worth be low? Well, confidence doesn't necessarily equate to self-worth. Confidence is believing in my *ability* to accomplish my goal. Repeated successes/achievements built that confidence and sustained it. However, my *need* for the constant pursuit of achieving was rooted in my low level of self-worth. Low self-worth shows up in different ways for different people. This was one of the ways it showed up for me. I had other ways too like my codependency and people-pleasing tendencies that I mentioned previously.

Are any coming up for you?

Please don't misunderstand and conclude that all beauty pageant contestants and high achievers have poor self-worth because that's not true. It's the why (the intent) behind what we are doing that gives us clues about our self-worth. If I was doing it to grow and expand and provide myself with varied life experiences, then that would have been a healthy "why."

But in my case, I equated achievement to being worthy. I needed the external admiration and all the hoopla because being in the spotlight in these various ways made me feel seen and significant. In reality, it was short-lived and left me feeling empty to then search for the *next* thing that would give me that fix.

So, being fertility challenged and not being able to achieve a baby majorly rocked my already poor and unstable sense of worth. I had already identified myself as becoming a mother (an aspiration/upcoming achievement I had as a youngster), so every failure in doing so made me feel less significant, less worthy, and unidentifiable in my eyes because my self-worth was wrapped up in achieving, and specifically the achievement of motherhood. The struggle I endured of working so hard to get pregnant was me trying to show my worth to God. *Look God, look how hard I am working! Don't I deserve to have a baby? What else do I need to do to show you?* When, all the while, He was waiting for me to recognize my inherent divine worth without needing to *do* anything to earn it.

When I don't see myself as worthy, I'm coming from a place of lack, not being enough, and feeling undeserving at my core. I try to make "good" on that through performing and achieving. But each time I fail at conceiving, I exacerbate this sense of unworthiness and bring about even more of it. Think about the emotional state that coincides with a sense of unworthiness. It puts you in that stress response state of fight or flight which we know by now is not conducive to conception. It puts you out of alignment.

A baby is love and abundance, and there I was sitting in lack and not loving myself. The. Complete. Opposite. That is majorly out of alignment. How was I going to bring/attract a baby to me from that place? Me being in a place of self-love, knowing my worth, and living my life from that centered, calm place would be totally in alignment for conceiving as well as for attaining other important desires in my life.

Therein lies the goal: Know your true worth and value; be your true and authentic self on a regular basis.

And I can tell you right now, the level of love we experience in our relationships is a direct reflection of how we feel about ourselves and treat ourselves. Your parenting experience will be significantly more enjoyable and accompanied by greater ease if your self-worth is at a high and stable place. So, let's see what we can do about that!

> There's a place in the soul where you've never been wounded.
>
> —Meister Eckhart

The Truth of Who You Are

Who are you?

How would you answer that?

Would you say, I am a nurse, a teacher, a waitress, or some other occupation? Or I am a sister, a daughter, an aunt, a wife?

These are labels, but they aren't *who* you are.

You *are not* **your thoughts.**

You are **the one** who thinks them.

You *are not* **your body.**

You are **the one** living inside your body.

You *are not* **your feelings.**

You are **the one** who feels your feelings.

You *are not* **your choices.**

You are **the one** who makes them.

That **one** is perfect in God's eyes. Our soul is the essence of who we are. This person, this **one**, is free of ego and attachments. Eckhart Tolle and many others teach that the essence of who we are when we are not thinking is our true selves, our consciousness. And this consciousness cannot in any way be defined by any outward or physical expression of us.

God created us; each and every one of us is an expression of Him, a holy concept breathed into existence. The profound reverence and respect that you have for God, you need to have for yourself. God doesn't make mistakes, only beauty. We are part of Him, and He dwells within us. With that knowing, you are complete and whole as you are, just by virtue of being here. This self is inherently worthy. You never need to do anything to earn His love for you. It is unconditional. It is vital for you to wrap your brain around this and take this in.

I mean think about it: out of 7.8 billion people in the world, there is no one—*not one*—just like you and YOU were chosen to be here, designed by God for a specific purpose. You are God's masterpiece, His unique work of art. You were perfectly created just as you are with your own unique gifts and talents that will be expressed in a way that only you can do. There is no need to prove your worth or value here. You are enough just as you are!

Our souls *know* this truth, but as I've mentioned before, we as babies and children are dependent on those around us so we can survive and thrive and, as a result, we adapt ourselves to *be* what we have learned will best get our needs met and meet cultural norms. This makes us veer further from our authentic self, our true self. Layers form over the top of that true essence which is our ego's way of protecting us, and we develop personas (ways of being) that help us get our needs met. We believe these personas are WHO WE ARE. Layers include roles like people pleaser, overachiever, bully, perfectionistic, martyr, workaholic, control freak, or cool/funny guy. We wear these masks to be perceived a certain way and to conform to specific societal/cultural standards in order to be accepted, feel loved, and belong. Without them we may not even know who we are because we are so conditioned to them. We have lost sight of our true essence—our true self—the one we are at our core beneath all the masks and layers. We forget that we are the perfect masterpiece that God created who is already worthy because we came from Him, the divine. As Christians, we are all part of the body of Christ and with that being the case, how can we not be enough?

In coming back to your true self and knowing who you are in Christ, it won't be through adding something to make that sink in. It will be in shedding (subtracting) all those layers (personas/masks) to reveal the essence of you. The shedding of the egoic defenses, the conditioning, the control, the emotional wounds, and the false beliefs about yourself and life. You will need to determine who you *aren't* to find who you *are*. When you can do that, you will experience a sense of *freedom* like no other.

This level of honor for yourself will show you that you don't need to achieve, conform, compromise yourself, perform, or act in any certain way to attain that worthiness. When you have truly internalized this knowing, and not just conceptually, but a knowing deep in your spirit, it won't really matter what someone else has that you don't. It won't really matter what their opinion of you is, and it won't really matter if someone disagrees with your point of view or lifestyle. You won't take things so personally. Rejection doesn't carry the same weight. People pleasing doesn't feel mandatory anymore. You won't feel like you need to judge or criticize others because you see the same unconditional sense of worth in them and respect their uniqueness. External validation isn't necessary anymore.

Your only comparison or competition is with yourself in becoming the best version of the human God created you to be, growing and maturing spiritually to become more and more like God's character. Although our essence is perfect, all that emanates from it in our human expression, such as our personality, physical traits/body, or abilities is imperfect. In claiming our worth, we accept and honor all these parts of ourselves, flaws and all. You honor and love the way God created you because there was purpose and love behind it.

Having a high degree of self-love doesn't mean that you believe you are superior to anyone else, it means that you don't view anyone else as superior to you either. No human being is more worthy than another. Self-love is not being cocky, conceited, or arrogant. True authenticity is a quiet, humble confidence and knowing. This self-love sets the stage for every other relationship in your life to be at its peak. Your relationships become a place of giving and not getting or taking because you are full within yourself and don't need to be filled up by others. It is in the giving that we receive anyway. What we *are*—how we show up in this world and what we put out there—comes back to us. That is true fulfillment.

We are so busy being who we think we need to be to get the love we want from others to reaffirm we are okay, and guess what? We already *are* okay and enough. So, enough of that!

We all need love and connection. These are basic needs, but it's important to get those needs met within yourself first. As an adult, you are responsible for feeling whole, fulfilled, and complete within yourself and not putting that responsibility onto someone else. When you know that you are enough and honor and respect yourself, then you don't *need* a spouse/partner. You don't *need* to be a mother. Yes, we are a social species and God created us to enjoy these connections to enhance our lives and expand our joy. But let those connections be a choice, not a requirement; let them supplement your existence and not *be* your existence. Then, these relationships are a bonus and your desire for them comes from a pure loving place as opposed to a needy place. This allows you to *fully* love others. It's pure and unconditional and doesn't require that they (or some acquired possession or goal attainment) make you happy. This perspective upgrades your life experience, and those connections will be healthy ones because you don't require getting your needs met through them.

I can remember saying to myself so many times, *I **have** to be a mom*. That desperation, that neediness, invoked fear and distress within me as the years went by. If I had felt complete and whole without having to hold the title of mother, the experience of being fertility challenged wouldn't have been as painful for me emotionally.

Would I have still had the desire to be a mother? Yes.

Would I have been disappointed that it wasn't happening? Absolutely.

But it wouldn't have consumed me and put me in such a state of distress as I struggled to find my worth and who I really was, if I couldn't be a mother. I would have already been secure in the knowledge of my worth and "enoughness."

Consequently, that peace of mind, body, and spirit and the energy emanating from me—that inner state of being—would have reflected in my external world and been in alignment for conception to occur. Amazing, right? I got in my own way. I hope you are getting this and can apply it to your own situation.

Imagine you are at a big party or a networking event. God is there. He sees you and you lock eyes. He approaches you and whisks you away to introduce you to guests.

He says, "Meet (insert your name). She is absolute true love. She makes people smile just by being next to her. She is my beloved. She is a shining light to all and my precious treasure. She is a beautiful symphony that I composed note by note. She is passion, purpose, love, incredible, and priceless."

Whew! What an introduction!

Now, if you could see yourself that way, the way God sees you, in truth, there would be no lack, fear, or confusion, only an abundance of love, appreciation, gratitude, and trust.

How do you learn to take on this view if you haven't seen yourself as worthy for most of your life? How do you shift this underlying feeling of being undeserving that may have been in the backdrop of your life even without your awareness of it, and that also might be keeping your baby at bay?

Well, I can tell you what I did to raise my level of self-worth. I had to keep reminding myself of my worth. I started approaching my life with this change in thinking. I figured out where my poor self-worth stemmed from and how I allowed it to continue to play out in my life. It's a work in progress and it didn't shift overnight. I also didn't do it alone. I enlisted the help of several knowledgeable mentors, and I did the inner work over the course of several years.

Inner child work was a big piece of my inner work because it involves self-exploration and dissecting personality dynamics that were created from unmet emotional/psychological or physical needs in childhood that are carried into adulthood which can have a profound impact on our life. We act from our unhealed wounds. The inner child is the child (little self) that lives within the psyche. The inner child also represents the innocent, playful, creative, and awe-like wonder we have toward life that we still need to nurture. We really are just children who have aged in that we carry into adulthood our conditioning and belief systems that were formed in our early childhood years. We continue to see ourselves through this lens and make life decisions based on it until we dig into those beliefs, challenge them, and reveal what's true for us now. Doing this work helped me to grow so much as a person.

I became aware of my patterns, beliefs, and conditioning to better understand myself, and I made changes in those areas that would better serve me. Then, I stepped into my life from this place, took some risks, and then the proof was in the pudding, so to speak. That meant risking disappointing or displeasing others and in doing so realizing that I didn't lose the connection with them after all. I gained respect for myself and a sense of inner peace because I didn't sacrifice myself or abandon my true self for the approval of someone else. I was in my integrity and that peaceful feeling is priceless. I value myself enough, regardless of how it turns out, to take that step in the first place. I'm human and flawed, so at times I slip back; however, I am conscious of it, and I reset. I get back in the saddle again because the rewards are many. Is my self-worth perfect now? No, but that isn't the goal. We can't be perfect. But my self-worth is at a healthy place and continues to expand.

Your true self is constantly evolving as you continue to learn, improve, and grow in your understanding of yourself in relation to the world you live in.

You need to try it out, and in doing so, you'll find that the results are so much more in your favor and those around you in the long run because it comes from a place of love when you do it with good intention.

You will need to talk *to* yourself more than you *listen* to yourself. Speak truth to yourself and don't listen to any of your stinking thinking and limiting beliefs. You get to believe whatever you want, but the truth is *You are worthy*. Period.

Make this your mantra:

I am 100 percent lovable and worthy by God's design and this truth is aligned in my thoughts, words, and actions.

This chapter is just to whet your appetite in this area and bring your attention to the power it holds in your life. I recognize that this may not be something you can change easily or quickly on your own. But it certainly is a starting place and, with this awareness you now have, it gets the ball rolling. A qualified coach or a counselor can greatly assist you with this. When I coach clients, I help them gain awareness and clarity in this area because we aren't always able to see all on our own how we have been getting in our own way. We are on autopilot with engrained addictive patterns of thinking and behaving.

Getting To Know You

When you are being your true self, you feel calm, centered, at peace, and emotionally stable. It's important to be aware of what being in this space feels like, so you are better able to distinguish between when you are in that authentic place and in your integrity as opposed to operating from your conditioned habitual ways that don't serve you well.

I'm going to describe to you how to access that place, your true self, where you can tap into the spirit of Christ within you, where peace, joy, and love reside, where God dwells. This place can also be referred to as your higher self because when we are here, we are most like God because He *is* these attributes. This place of centered presence allows you to hear the still quiet voice within where God speaks to you. That intuitive knowing that comes from this place is God speaking to us through the Holy Spirit. God is always talking to us. We just don't quiet ourselves and our minds enough to listen and hear Him.

This place is where we surrender our minds and drop into our heart. There is no anxiety, fear, or worry in this space because it can't compete with love and peace. When you do this simple practice on a regular basis, you will become familiar with this feeling and, therefore, be able to discern when you are being your true self in all areas of your life because you have this as a reference point. It's in this place that you will find the answers you need. It's where you should make decisions from because you have clarity here. You are clear minded and not in an emotionally charged state.

Being your true self, your whole self—where your mind, body, and soul are aligned—is where you want to be as much as possible because only good comes from this. Certainly, you will feel all other emotions, but use those feelings as messengers indicating what you need to pay attention to in your life. Fully be with the feeling and determine what needs to shift or be adjusted, and then *do* it. Then, you'll be reset to that place of peace. Your true self should be your home base and what runs the show in your life, rather than your ego. Your ego has its place, but it shouldn't be in the driver's seat.

God is love and peace. He is within us and when we seek Him from this place, we cultivate self-love and peace. We have all we need within us. I feel so empowered from this place because I am calm, at peace, my body is relaxed, and I am open to guidance in my life. It's my strength and I am in my personal power through Christ within me and working through me. This place of peace and love is where He wants us to be. It is our greatest challenge, but the place from which we receive the greatest blessings.

In my many years of struggling to conceive, I was not my true, authentic self. How do I know? Because I wasn't at peace. I was clinging to an outcome I believed *had* to happen and I was controlling it in every way I could imagine in order to have it come to fruition. It was stressful, exhausting, and dishonoring to myself, my body, and to God. Definitely not peaceful or loving. When we aren't *that*, we are out of alignment.

So, let's go into our heart space.

Seek out a place that is free of distractions and interruptions. Sit in an upright position as you would to prepare for prayer or meditation. Close your eyes and place your hands over your heart. God is as near to you as your heartbeat. Take a long and slow breath in through your nose from deep in your belly, not just from your chest. Hold it for a few seconds and then exhale slowly through your mouth. Do this several times. You will feel the relaxation in your body. Keep up this slow and steady breathing.

As you breathe in, imagine breathing in peace. Become aware of the presence of God within and your oneness with Him. It may feel as though you are even breathing in and out from your heart space.

Stay with it. This is where you will feel the love that God has filled you with. As you continue breathing and holding your hands on your heart, in your mind say, *I am here with you*. If a thought comes into your awareness, just acknowledge it, and let it go without letting the thought take you away with it. Do this for as long as you wish. It may be five minutes or twenty, stay with it. You can even ask God a question you desire guidance on before you start or ask it once you are in this relaxed state. Sometimes I will also say, *I AM Peace. I AM Love. I AM Wisdom.*

You may get an answer to your question during this prayerful heart-centered time, or He may lead you to it via another manner by speaking through someone else in your circle of influence, a word in scripture, information put at your fingertips, or even through nature.

What you experienced during this is what self-love feels like and is. Self-love is really receiving God's love. You are made in the image and likeness of God, and you need to treat yourself as the divine being that you are. It is loving yourself *as you are*, imperfections, flaws, and all. It's loving yourself even with this physical body limitation that is present with your not becoming pregnant. Do not focus on what your body isn't doing for you. Focus on the miracle that your body truly is and look at all it is designed to do. It's only going to be healed by the love you give it.

We don't usually pour love into areas of our body that don't function optimally. Usually, we have anger and frustration that it's not working efficiently. Imagine the healing light of God flooding every cell of your being and every corner of your mind. Be completely open to God's healing energy. When you are present in your heart-centered time, you are in your most receptive state. Allow God to guide you about your fertility challenges from your higher self when you are in your heart space. Ask God for your next steps. Make decisions from this place and not your lower stress response self. Seek God first before others. Meet Him here and He can show you how to let go of the things that are holding you back from your blessings. Ask Him to show you what He needs you to see with this situation in your life.

Do not blame yourself for your condition, piling on guilt and shame with thoughts like, *Maybe I shouldn't have been on the pill so many years* or *Maybe I partied too much* or *Maybe I'm being punished for sinful past decisions I made* and so forth. Look for the opportunity this situation is giving you, the opportunity to transform many areas of your life. Have compassion and love for yourself. That is what heals. This is a steppingstone to something greater in your life if you awaken to this and allow it to be. It is a chance to upgrade your whole self, body, mind, and soul, to prepare you to be a great parent and better prepared for all facets of your life. Coming from this healthier, aligned place will help you to achieve your desired outcomes.

This fertility challenge is here to help you. Use every bit of it to your advantage and you will thrive through it to a better, more fully developed version of yourself than when you entered it.

When you know who you are in Christ and know your worth, you trust that He will deliver your highest good. You have faith in that and then there is no need for fear, worry, doubt, or questioning. You can live in that joy and peace despite your circumstances. Sometimes we *think* we know what is best for us, but God is the only one who really knows. We don't want what isn't best for us, so we need to trust Him and His timing for our life.

As you can tell from my self-disclosure in the past few chapters, I have actually had quite a few missing pieces to the fertility challenge puzzle: surrender, story, emotional state, self-worth.

How about you? What are the missing pieces that you are finding?

The good news is that once you find them, you can work on shifting them to achieve your desired outcomes. That's what I did and continue to do. You hold the power to do that which is so incredibly awesome! You hold the lock, and you hold the key. Claim your power and own your greatness!

Self-care is another way we love ourselves and demonstrate the respect and honor we have for ourselves. We can only give to others in proportion to what we give ourselves. The fuller we are, the more able we are to give to others from that full cup. If we are self-deprecating and not taking care of ourselves to the point that we are depleted energy-wise and approaching burnout, what are we really giving to others? Not our best, that's for sure.

The level of love and compassion you have for yourself is the barometer for what you can offer others. The thing is, we don't do what we need to do for ourselves if we don't view ourselves as worthy. Do you see how everything emanates from this core knowing of our inherent worth? That, in and of itself, makes it clear that having a strong sense of self-worth would move your *star* on our infamous scale toward the direction of baby success and away from stress and suffering.

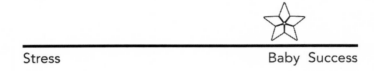

Stress   Baby Success

In the following chapter, we will cover specific ways that you can show yourself that level of self-care to keep your tank full in addition to many other action steps you can take to move you further down the path to motherhood.

Reflections and Journal Prompts

What do you believe about yourself? Take your time with this one.

How would you rate your level of self-worth currently? How would you rate it for the majority of your life?

How does your level of self-worth show up for you in your life? Refer to the list in the beginning of the chapter to assist you.

What do you love about yourself?

What do others love about you and admire you for?

What makes you unique and special?

Read this list often.

Find a childhood photo of yourself between the ages of four and six. Look at this precious little you. How would you talk to this little girl when she is scared, lonely, unsure of herself, in need of love and attention, and wants to be seen and accepted for who she is? Is that how you talk to yourself typically? Keep this photo displayed nearby to serve as a reminder to treat yourself lovingly and with compassion and forgiveness. Write what you love most about yourself on the back of the photo.

What did you do today that you are proud of yourself for?

How can you love yourself more right now? What is the most loving thing you can do for yourself in this moment?

Chapter Seven
Strategy

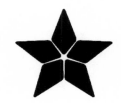

Enjoy where you are on the way to where you are going.

—Joyce Meyer

My intent with this book is for you to have tools in your arsenal to help you maximize your chances of conception and achieve your dream of motherhood. It is also my hope that as you implement what you discover about yourself along the way, it will ease your emotional pain and suffering during your journey.

So far in each chapter, I have been bringing to your attention significant factors that may be playing a part in your fertility challenges. Your job is to gain an understanding of them and to reflect on how they impact your personal situation. Awareness is the first step toward change. Once you have that and can identify what needs to shift, you need a plan of action to optimally address what requires change. This we will call *strategy* and that is what this chapter is all about. We certainly have covered some strategies in the prior chapters already; however, this chapter is solely devoted to it and will provide you with a succinct framework you can easily reference that will be incredibly valuable to you.

What's in the way of getting what you want? One of the ways this book assists you in closing the gap between where you are and what you want is by implementing my five-point tool. This chapter actually finishes off the fifth point of the Five-Point SuperStar System, and I'm going to demonstrate to you now how to use it as its own strategy.

Going clockwise: Top point (Surrender), Point 2 (Story), Point 3 (State), Point 4 (Self), Point 5 (Strategy)

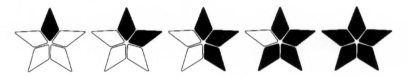

Each point of the star signifies one of the factors (puzzle pieces) that may be potentially blocking your baby blessing. Each point of the star has a chapter devoted to it—four of which we have covered already. This five-point star is an extremely useful strategy in its own right. You use it to answer the question, *What is in the way of getting what I want?* This is what we have been doing in the preceding chapters with you uncovering your missing piece or pieces. You determine those and then take respective action steps.

Incidentally, this tool will be highly beneficial to you in *any* area of your life that is not where you would like it to be such as career, marriage, finances, family relationships, friendships, physical health, or whatever you may be struggling with and is weighing you down. This star will be a useful mnemonic device for you to access at any point to help you determine what is getting in the way of what you want and then apply it to that situation. I made it simple and user friendly by having each point begin with the letter "s" just like the word *star*.

A star is a shining light, just like each of us has our own light that we shine as a unique expression of God. We shine our brightest when all points of this star are in alignment. We illuminate brightly when we are our true selves and live authentically, when we know our true worth, when we are open, present, and allow life to unfold, and when our thoughts and emotions are in sync with all of that. It is then that we are living our life as the SuperStar we were designed to be. When one or more of these points are out of alignment, our light dims and sometimes we get swallowed up into the darkness with our lives going down a path of pain and suffering that can be hard to find our way out of.

Let this star be your way out of the darkness, your GPS so to speak. As you address the points of the star that have dimmed, the positive shifts that occur within you and in your life will brighten to full force. It will guide you out of the darkness and heaviness toward joy, peace, love, and a fulfilling life. When one of these points is off-kilter and it puts you out of alignment, you will know it because you won't feel at peace. Use the star to assess what's contributing to the issue at hand and apply the strategy(ies) to get back in alignment. Perhaps you'll find that you need to change your perspective of the situation (story), or maybe you have been suppressing your feelings and displacing them on others (state), or maybe you have been burning the candle at both ends and doing it from an empty cup because your self-care has been virtually non-existent, and your cup needs some filling (self). Maybe it's time to rest your mind from trying to figure everything out all the time and trust that things are unfolding in divine timing and for your highest good (surrender).

This star (and all that it represents) can help you coach yourself to thinking better, feeling better, and living the life you want to live. Let this shining star be your light guide. The contents of each star point serve as stepping stones illuminating your way out of the darkness and into the brightest light. In doing so, you shine your personal God-given light as it was meant, and the ripple effect of this impacts all around you in the most positive way.

The star is a framework that can serve as a starting point for you. It is a great self-awareness tool to help you size up the situation and it enables you to take a 30,000 foot. view so you can use the specific strategies that will target what's getting in the way of living your best life. Using the star tool in partnership with a life coach or therapist, as I do with my clients, can be valuable to help you dig deep to the root of what's going on, keep you accountable to what you are committed to working on, and keep you moving forward. A decision to do this is a sign of self-respect, courage, and empowerment, and not one of weakness.

So, mama-to-be, what is it that you want? What is your heart's deepest desire right now?

I think you shouted, "TO HAVE A BABY!!!!"

I hear you loud and clear and so does God. So, then let's get to that Strategy point of your SuperStar.

Let's keep it simple and clear so you can implement it with certainty.

This strategy I am about to share will serve as your umbrella (main) strategy that all others will fall under. Keep this strategy at the forefront of your mind as the main approach.

Do your best and let God do the rest.

Or another way we can say it so it is even more specific to your desire would be:

I prime the pump and God creates the bump or trumps it.

Your priming the pump *is* your **doing your part**, i.e., doing what you have control over, which entails putting into practice and truly embodying what will set you up best to create the most fertile environment for conception to occur. The rest, which is out of your control, is up to God to do His way and in His timing. **Trumps it** refers to God having something better planned for you than your mind can even imagine if your prayer isn't answered specifically to your request.

TheFreedictionary.com defines *prime the pump* as action that encourages the growth of something or helps it to succeed. **Priming the pump** is doing specifically what will best create a fertile environment. Doing your part to relax your body and heal the system so it can do what it is innately designed to do so that you may *stop doing* what works against that and *do* what promotes that. Doing *that* will, in fact, be doing your best.

We have discussed before that when you are healthy and consistently aligned in body, mind, and spirit, your body is fertile, barring any major anatomical issues that would make it impossible, such as not having a uterus or your partner has no sperm at all (azoospermia), or something along those lines. You create the conditions and environment for conception to occur. Therefore, the goal is having you be fit and healthy in those three areas of body, mind, and spirit bringing you back to that place of wholeness because it is just unbalanced right now.

So, we become *fit* in each of these areas by priming the pump in each of them. You have already begun priming the pump if you have been doing the suggested work in the previous chapters. This chapter contains more ways to prime the pump. Please do not overwhelm yourself thinking that you need to put everything listed in this chapter in place. You will need to discern from them which ones will be most beneficial to your priming your pump. Small, meaningful shifts can be very transformative.

When you want to achieve something, it's best to learn and follow suit from those who have had success in that which you wish to achieve. Now, by no means are they doing everything "right" all the time. Because, as we know, many of them still conceive despite not always making the healthiest choices for their bodies. However, their bodies are in alignment enough that conception happens. So, since we fall in the category of being the underdogs, we need to do what's ideal (not perfect) so it's *more than enough* to compensate for how far off balance we may be, so that we can turn things around.

Let's tackle this.

You want to *achieve* motherhood.

How would you say that a great (not perfect) mom behaves most of the time?

How does she show up for her child?

How does she view herself?

What is her emotional state most of the time?

How does the mom that you hope to be live her life?

Take a moment to think about that.

I would describe the ideal mom in this way: loving, compassionate, nurturing, emotionally regulated/calm/stable, not self-absorbed, patient, present, giving, centered, knows her own worth, and is aware/intentional.

This is my ideal. Can we achieve this 100 percent of the time? Of course not. We are human. But we are going to aim high to achieve success. Were your descriptors similar to mine? How often would you say you have been demonstrating these characteristics lately? How many of them? Any of them? Remember we discussed that our inner world is reflected in our outer world. Let's get you showing up in your life like those traits on your list most of the time. Then we are in business!! Keeping it simple, **you need to "be"** (embody) **what you want to be** (a mother). Live from the place of having already received your desire. Act as if it's a done deal. Trust that it is on its way. This enables you to be at rest.

"Being" it now is what will provide a fertile environment to conceive your baby as well as the ideal conditions for it to grow and develop in. Even gestationally, babies absorb the energy (your emotional state) of the mother. The mother's biochemistry has a direct impact on the baby through the umbilical cord. The baby picks up stress hormones in the womb. A baby's DNA and cells respond to the environment they are provided. So, doing this on the front end—being intentional about being in that calm, regulated energy space—is a gift to yourself and your baby.

The fertile woman isn't thinking about getting pregnant all the time. It doesn't consume her and her life. She is open and in flow with life, not controlling and clinging to it having to happen and NOW! This keeps her body out of stress mode and in alignment. She has a trusting expectancy that it *will* happen and doesn't need to perseverate on it. She just goes about her life. In this way, she embodies many of the traits we listed above. She is present (not worrying about the future), she is calm and centered, and she isn't self-absorbed. You may be thinking, *But how do I stop thinking about it all the time?* No worries, there are more strategies to come that will help you do just that. This thinking about it all the time has become a pattern. Patterns can be changed and substituted with new patterns, ones that move you in the direction of your heart's deepest desire.

The key is getting you to relax your body, mind, and spirit, and to bring it all back in alignment to complete wholeness so your body can do what it was innately designed to do. I believe this may be the reason why the majority of ART procedures are unsuccessful because science alone can't offset an imbalanced system. *All areas* need to be addressed, not just the body.

Approximately 2 percent of infants born in the US every year are conceived using ART (CDC's Fertility Clinic Success Rate Report, 2018). In 2020, there were 3,613,647 infants born in the US (Centers for Disease Control and Prevention, National Vital Statistics System, 2020). When you do the math, that would mean approximately 72,272 of them were a result of ART. That 2 percent figure represents only the successful ART. How many procedures fail? The 2018 summary data representing all IVF clinics in the United States, published by the Society for Assisted Reproductive Technologies, or SART, show that about 47 percent of couples who undergo IVF treatment will achieve a pregnancy and have at least one child as a result of their treatment, provided that the female partner is less than thirty-five years old and uses her own eggs rather than donated eggs. So, doing the math, 47 percent achieve pregnancy using ART, which means 53 percent fail. That summary data also indicated that when the female partner is forty-one to forty-two years of age, the success rate of achieving pregnancy through ART drops to about 10 percent. I know when I was in your shoes, I didn't research the success rate of it. I was hell-bent on doing whatever I could to conceive, so I was just happy it existed as an option, not realizing that the chance of failure was rather high. Let's improve the success rates of these procedures and, perhaps, minimize the need for them in general, by putting into practice what is contained in this book.

What's beautiful about this approach is that these strategies give you a sense of control in creating the effect you are looking for with them, which is body, mind, and spirit alignment to help facilitate conception. These choices you make will get you that result if you are consistent with them. That's empowering. That's very different from all the overwhelm of not being sure which way to go next and being at the mercy of the minimal success of the complicated and expensive ART process. The role that the whole being (body/mind/spirit) plays regarding fertility issues is typically not factored into the equation, which is catastrophic. So, putting your focus on regaining your wholeness will allow you to reap many rewards, one of which may just be your baby.

Mind

Let's start with the mind. Chapter Four—Story gave you some great ideas in this area, but let's take it further.

To embody that which you desire (to be fertile), what kind of thoughts would promote that? What kind of self-talk? What would conversation topics be like with others? What would you need to believe? What would you focus on? Is it different from what you typically do?

It is so important that you consciously think about what you *want* to experience and not on what you aren't experiencing. Instead of thinking this:

I'm the only one in my friend group that doesn't have children. What if it never happens for me?

Think this:

I will become a mother at the right time for me.

This shift is profound.

Thinking about what you want to experience can take the form of visualization, vision boards, positive affirmations, mantras, prayers, quoting/declaring scripture, gratitude, and faith.

Picture yourself in your mind's eye as already having reached your goal with your baby in your arms. This is called visualization. Let your brain know what is important by focusing on the details of what you want. It will get the RAS working in your favor. What we imagine can affect our physiology in a major way, for better or for worse.

Just take this simple example of visualizing a lemon. Picture a lemon in your mind's eye, a nice vibrant yellow. Picture holding it in your hand, placing it on a cutting board, and then taking a knife and cutting the lemon in half. Take one-half of the lemon up to your mouth and lick it. Now, do you notice yourself salivating a little bit? Incredible, right? The power of the mind. The amazing mind-body connection.

How can we use this to help you?

Close your eyes and create a mental picture of you being pregnant and giving birth. Use all your senses to enhance the vividness of the image in your mind. How does your baby look (hair/no hair, what color)? How does your baby smell? Feel the softness of her skin. How does he feel lying against your chest? Can you hear her little breaths or little gurgles she makes? What would it feel like to look into your baby's eyes as you hold him in your arms? What is the sensation? Think about it in a relaxed and cheerful way.

Stay with it. Breathe it in. Say out loud, "I AM a mother." We've discussed before about the energy of the two words (I AM) being extremely potent, so what you put after them is as well. You are claiming this. Your mind, body, and spirit are in unison with this exercise. This only takes a few minutes, but it is very powerful. Do this each morning upon waking and in bed before you fall asleep each night. Do it a minimum of thirty consecutive days so it becomes a habit.

You can also create healing in your body through visualization. Envision your body being *receptive* to fertilization and it actually taking place. Envision your body healthy and whole and couple it with affirmations.

I am open and ready to receive.

I am whole.

I am love.

My body is receptive to receive and nurture life.

The body manifests what the mind nurtures. Make this one a habit as well.

Perhaps you are thinking, *But I do think about conceiving and how great it will be to be a mother.* Hmmm, well the trick to this is that alignment thing we keep referring to. It's the thoughts that we *think the most* with the *most conviction* backed up with our words and deeds that show up in our lives. You may have had those thoughts, but they weren't your most prominent ones, so they were overcome by those with more conviction and were solidified with your words and actions.

Let's back up your baby visualizations with congruent words, attitude, and actions. First, when you picture yourself pregnant and giving birth, follow it up with the words, "Thank you God. Thank you for making me a mom." You are recognizing this blessing as it is and with no doubt whatsoever. You believe it first in your mind and heart, so that you see it in your reality. *This* is having the thought process of already having attained what you want. That means, and I say this with so much love, you are going to stop talking about *the problem*, which is **I can't get pregnant**. Stop talking about not being able to get pregnant. Stop thinking about it. Stop beating yourself up about it. Stop wishing it would be different. That's the REAL problem. We are shifting your thoughts through this process. We are shifting your focus to be on *your passion of being a mom*, instead of *your fear of not being a mom*. That's huge!

Mantras and positive affirmations can serve as "pattern interrupts" for those fear-based thoughts that don't serve you well and have been on autopilot for a while. These rewire your brain in the same way it was programmed with the fear-based thoughts, through repetition linked with emotion. Your brain will accept these new thoughts as fact.

Here are some that you can use:

I am worthy.

I choose how I think, feel, and react to life.

I know something good can happen at any moment.

I am joyful as I go about my day.

I am a blessing to all who cross my path.

I am an example of love in the words I choose to speak today.

I am healed.

I am fertile.

I will mother the child I am meant to mother in divine timing.

I choose peace.

My focus is the next step, not the entire path.

I am kind and gentle to myself.

I love my miraculous body.

I am in the flow of divine order.

Becoming a mother is so easy.

I am nurtured, loved, and supported.

Feel free to also come up with some of your own. These can be written on sticky notes and placed all around your house. Put your favorite one as a screen saver on your computer or on the home screen of your phone to keep these thoughts at the forefront of your mind.

Belief is nearly everything. Look at the many studies that have been done for drug effectiveness testing and the placebo effect was in full force. To explain how the placebo effect can play out, let's say there is a clinical trial to test the effectiveness of a particular drug. Patients are randomly placed in one of two groups. In the first group (test group), 100 patients are given the actual drug to relieve targeted symptoms and in the second group (control group), 100 patients are given a placebo (a sugar pill in essence that looks like the drug being tested) but are *told* they are receiving the drug being tested. In the first test group, 75 of the 100 reported that they felt better. In the second control group, the results were basically the same even though they didn't receive the drug.

Why?

Belief.

Belief itself shifts biology.

Those in the second test group believed they were getting the drug and expected that it would help. They surrendered to this belief and relaxed in it. Pretty powerful. You may find it fascinating to do your own research on documented studies that demonstrate the placebo effect.

Be a Vibrational Match to That Which You Desire

Now, let's work on embodying the energy and emotional state that will be congruent with this mindset shift. As your thoughts shift, your emotional state shifts along with them. Your goal is to be in the emotional energy state of that which you want to achieve. Where are you putting your mental/emotional energy? It needs to be in the joy of being a mother, looking forward to it, being in the emotional state of what you will feel like when you are one. What will you *feel* like when you get the call that you are pregnant or see that positive pregnancy test result? What will it *feel* like to get the ultrasound picture of your baby and hear his heartbeat? What will it *feel* like to celebrate this at your *own* baby shower? These feelings you are identifying for yourself right now is where you need to make a *conscious* effort to be *most* of the time. It is *that inner state* that will be matched in your outer world.

Do not allow yourself to be on autopilot with fear-based thoughts like *I don't know how much longer I can take this* or *What if this round of IVF doesn't work?* or *I don't know what I'll do if I get my period again this month.* It may seem like you are thinking about conceiving, but the energy behind this is fear, anxiety, frustration, sadness, and desperation, coming from a place of lack. Thinking about how you can rid yourself of these fertility issues, obsessing about how to fix them, and worrying about whether more failure is coming your way is a heavy, low energy state. This *is not* the inner state that you want matched in your outer world, so shift it. You get to choose the emotional energy instead of allowing it to control you because you are very aware now that you hold the power to do this! And you do it with the strategies we just discussed and will continue to discuss in this chapter to keep your state in a high place.

Doing your visualizations, mantras, and affirmations regularly and really feeling the emotions of them will help get you there. You can also bump it up a few notches by actively pursuing and participating in activities that produce those feelings of joy, bliss, elation, happiness, love, and contentment.

What can you do that will create those feelings? These are also great forms of self-care incidentally. For me it's playing tennis, painting, reading, snuggling with my dogs, singing/dancing to my favorite songs, sipping a pumpkin spice latte, or watching a favorite sitcom.

Come up with your own list and make selections from it each day. Having these feelings become your emotional set point is what we are striving for. Setting your phone alarm at different points of the day for emotional state check-ins is a simple and convenient way to keep your emotional awareness level at a good place so you can make changes accordingly. Also, refer to Chapter Ten, which is on happiness, to assist you more with this.

We now have you *thinking* like the mom you plan to be, *feeling* like her, and now your *actions* need to demonstrate that as well. Taking these actions is continuing to prepare for what you have asked for when there isn't the slightest bit of it in sight and having absolute faith—and proving it—in how you show up and in the choices you make.

If you truly believed this baby of yours was on its way to you, what would you be doing that is aligned with that?

You would go about your life freely, just as you did before you were trying to conceive, only in a more *conscious* way, more aware and intentional about your thoughts and emotional state. You would stop all the obsessive Google searching/symptom checking. You would stop forcing sex to happen and doing anything that feels "heavy" to you that tends to create panic, desperation, or stress.

Instead, focus on preparing for this baby in a balanced way. Perhaps you create a baby registry or create/refine your baby name ideas list. Get excited and creative about how you will design the baby nursery and start collecting design ideas. This kind of research is in the direction of where you want to be, and it feels fun and much lighter than the typical research you might have been doing to become pregnant. That's a great emotional state to promote.

Write a letter to your baby from the perspective of being so excited to meet her soon and be her mommy. Read it often. Here is an example of the one that I wrote and now keep in her baby album.

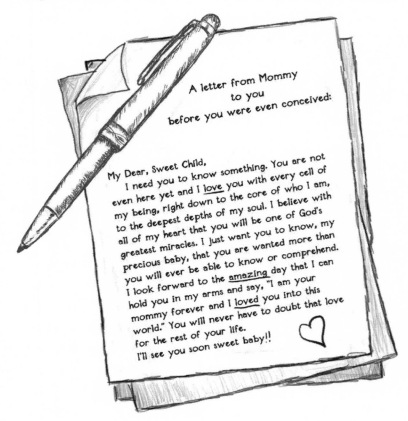

A letter from Mommy
to you
before you were even conceived:

My Dear, Sweet Child,
I need you to know something. You are not even here yet and I love you with every cell of my being, right down to the core of who I am, to the deepest depths of my soul. I believe with all of my heart that you will be one of God's greatest miracles. I just want you to know, my precious baby, that you are wanted more than you will ever be able to know or comprehend. I look forward to the amazing day that I can hold you in my arms and say, "I am your mommy forever and I loved you into this world." You will never have to doubt that love for the rest of your life.
I'll see you soon sweet baby!!

See the original letter on yourfertilityangel.com

You can even take part in activities that aren't necessarily baby focused but still symbolize the expectation of new life occurring. Plant a garden or even seeds in flowerpots to serve as a tangible reminder of life emerging and filling you with hope.

Gratitude

Be intentional about being grateful. Being intentional about looking for what is going well in your life and what you do appreciate and find beauty in will bring more of that to you in your life. Remember what we put our focus on grows and expands. Even in our complaints of the typical annoyances of life, we can find something to be grateful for. Pay attention to what you complain about. You hear yourself say, "This traffic is a nightmare!" With an attitude of gratitude, you now say, "I am grateful I have a safe and reliable car to drive." Or you hear yourself say, "I hate cooking and coming up with meal ideas all the time." Now, you say," I am blessed to have healthy food to eat and enjoy with others." You get the idea.

We need to find joy in what we already have in order to create the space to receive more. When you make this a regular practice to seek out and recognize what is beautiful and positive in your life, you begin to naturally focus on these blessings, and you crowd out those worrisome thoughts. It's impossible to be thankful and unhappy at the same time. Don't underestimate the power of this practice. Research shows when you are in a gratitude state regularly, it nourishes your nervous system and keeps you regulated. Create a habit of starting and/or ending your day reflecting on three things you were grateful for that day. I invite you to record them in your journal. When you have one of those *really* tough days, reading them will come in handy. Gratitude is a huge emotional state booster!

Be a Blessing

While you are waiting for your miracle, be a miracle to someone else. This condition can make us so self-absorbed with our grief, self-pity, jealousy, and obsession over how to turn it around, that we continue to downward spiral emotionally. We have a one-track mind for the most part. Being a blessing to someone else gets the focus off *you* and onto someone else. It's a great mindset shift and pattern interrupt. As you bless others, you are blessed. It's a win/win because you will bring joy to someone else by your action and to yourself through the satisfaction and pleasure you feel in serving another person in that way.

Who in your life needs something you can provide? What would absolutely make their day? What could you do to make this person's life easier or better today? It doesn't necessarily need to cost money and you may not even have to leave your house to do it.

You could send a thoughtful note to uplift or encourage a relative. You could send a text to a dear friend expressing how much you value your friendship. You could run an errand or do a chore your partner typically takes responsibility for and surprise him. You could drop off a home cooked meal to an elderly neighbor or invite him over for one. It might even be choosing not to nag or criticize your spouse the entire day.

Be creative in how you can give of yourself to others: your talent, your love, your attention, your money, your time. The thought you put behind deciding *who* it will be and *what* you will do for them will productively take your focus off your own stuff and use that energy for good. Can you imagine what this would do for you if you challenged yourself to come up with one person daily to bless? How do *you* want to be cared for during this trying time in your life? Go and do *that* for someone else. You will reap what you sow.

Body

Although I do have these strategies grouped into separate categories of mind, body, and spirit, be aware that many of them overlap one another, particularly due to the very nature that the body, mind, and spirit are so connected in general.

The body naturally knows what to do to heal itself. We just need to make it easier for it to do its job, not harder. That's the priming the pump part. Don't forget or minimize how important the following lifestyle basics are to keeping your body in a state of homeostasis. They are so basic, but so many of us don't prioritize these. They are foundational as a form of self-care as well.

The first is sleep. Ideally you should get between seven and nine hours of sleep each night. In this relaxed state, the body works to repair damage from stress of different forms it incurred that day. Lack of sleep can even contribute to weight gain because it increases cortisol levels which in turn increase appetite and sugar cravings. Proper sleep helps the brain function for better memory, alertness, decision-making, reaction time, balance, and much more. Proper sleep regulates the immune system by working to keep inflammation at bay. Getting the right amount of sleep strengthens your heart and improves your mood and energy levels. Would you say you get the proper amount of sleep most days or could this use some attention from you?

The second is ensure that you get a clean, balanced, healthy diet. You could Google this one and be inundated with a menagerie of best approaches, but for our purposes, let's keep it simple. The goal is to provide your body with optimal nutrition and minimize the amount of toxins the body must eliminate. The more toxins, the more stress to the body. The more stress to the body, the more it puts you out of balance.

Consuming organic/antibiotic free meats, fruits, and vegetables is ideal to minimize toxins. Whole grains and healthy fats/oils like avocado, olive oil, nuts, and seeds should be a part of your diet while avoiding the bad ones like margarine, vegetable oils, and fried foods. Avoid products containing white flour, dairy, soy, refined sugar, processed foods, and sugary foods and beverages. Minimize your caffeine and alcohol consumption or eliminate it completely during this time.

Keeping yourself hydrated adequately is critical, so drink half of your body weight in ounces of water. If you weigh 140 pounds, you need to be drinking seventy ounces of water daily. Taking prenatal multivitamins daily and getting out in nature for some Vitamin D is essential to your daily routine. I could go into many more specifics, but if you are able to stick to what I laid out here most of the time, you are doing your body well. If you feel that your diet/lifestyle is really in need of an overhaul, consulting with a nutritionist, holistic practitioner, or naturopath could be very beneficial to streamline your needs and have some accountability in maintaining the changes. There may be specific vitamins, minerals, and nutrients your body is deficient in, and dietary supplements may be recommended for you.

The third great thing you can do for yourself and your baby is to get regular exercise. Focus on moving your body in some way every day. If you can vary what you do to increase your intensity level and include full body strength training exercises, all the better. Start where you are, continue to improve it, and keep going. Run up and down your staircase, jump rope, take brisk walks, play sports, dance like crazy to your favorite music, ride your bike, do push-ups, do jumping jacks, skip around the house, or do yoga. Do what works for you but do *something*. Rebounding on a rebounder is a great exercise that's fun and doesn't take a lot of time. It detoxes the lymphatic system and helps your body to detox naturally, which is paramount to hormonal balance. Exercise is not only healthy for your overall body, but it helps you sleep better and enhances your mood.

These three components, as well as the suggestions made earlier to put and keep you in a high emotional state, need to be non-negotiables every day. Make it a routine and prioritize it daily.

Minimizing/eliminating your exposure to environmental toxins that are found in food, water, cleaning products, cosmetics, plastic, and the air we breathe, as well as toxins found in heavy metals, can positively impact your health.

Another area to consider is the amount of exposure you and your spouse have to EMF (electromagnetic frequency) radiation from cell phones, computers, and cell towers. Male sperm count and sperm effectiveness can be dramatically impacted by EMF radiation. Being aware of this potentiality and making changes in routine use and placement of cell phones/computers can make a positive difference.

Practicing presence with conscious breathing exercises has many benefits to the body and our overall health, such as improved concentration, better sleep, easing anxiety, and strengthening immunity. Our breathing happens involuntarily and is influenced by our emotions, thoughts, environment, state of health, and energy output. When we are stressed or anxious, our breathing can become rapid and shallow. I love that we can make changes to our breathing to induce the effects that we want to experience. When you are consciously aware of your breathing, you can do it in a way that will produce calmness and relaxation. Doing this at specific intervals throughout the day can help to keep your body out of that fight or flight state. Remember, your body reacts to your life, to your emotional state, so give it a good one that will keep it healthy.

Using your diaphragm and not your chest, breathe in deeply and slowly through your nose for the count of four, hold your breath for four, and then exhale long and slowly through your mouth (with pursed lips) for the count of eight. You can use different number amounts than I indicated but aim for your exhale to be double the count of your inhale. When we are stressed, we inhale longer than we exhale, so to relax the body, we need to exhale longer than we inhale. Go ahead and give this a try now and feel the effects of it for yourself. Repeat it three times or more, if you wish. Our sympathetic nervous system kicks in the fight or flight response when our body perceives stress. This breathing technique activates the parasympathetic nervous system which is responsible for rest and digestion. It's one of my favorite things to do to get in a relaxed state quickly. Focusing on breathing in this way keeps you present-centered, which is helpful in maintaining a peaceful state.

Here are some complementary and alternative treatment options that you may choose to participate in that can address the role the body may be playing in your fertility challenges. Many of these approaches help to move/release emotional energy that gets stuck in the body and puts the body out of balance.

- Reiki
- Acupuncture
- Massage
- Chakra healing/balancing
- Chiropractic care
- Bioenergetic therapy

These practices can help to decrease stress levels as well as to clear and balance your energy fields to restore and strengthen your ability to self-heal. You can explore these further on your own if you want to learn more about how they may help to facilitate conception.

Spirit

The quality of our spiritual health contributes to our overall health in the same way that our physical health and our mental health does. Spiritual wellness comprises how you view the meaning (purpose) of life, your coping skills along with emotional stability, where you derive hope from (faith), and how you facilitate a sense of inner peace and contentment with your life situation.

Body, mind, and spirit affect one another, so having all three areas balanced is key. You know you are spiritually healthy when you feel that sense of inner peace. Grounding and centering yourself through meditation, mindfulness, and/or prayer are beautiful ways to foster presence, peace, love, tapping into your intuition or higher self, and emotional regulation. There's a plethora of grounding meditations, other various forms of meditation, and mindfulness exercises out there for you to explore so you can select those that resonate with you.

I can honestly say that I didn't have that feeling of inner peace for most of my journey to become a mother. This kept me majorly misaligned. It saddens me to say it because I had always felt I had a good and close relationship with God. I was raised Catholic and attended church weekly, was in several prayer groups, prayed to God regularly, and routinely declared scripture in line with being able to conceive and receive God's promises. I went through all the motions, but when push came to shove, clearly my faith wasn't where I needed it to be.

After my failed IVF, Bonnie, one of my very spirit-filled Christian friends had a conversation with me and said that although God had closed this door for me, He had something even better planned for me.

Ephesians 3:20 says, "Now to Him Who, by (in consequence of) the [action of His] power that is at work within us, is able to [carry out His purpose and] do superabundantly, far over and above all that we [dare] ask or think [infinitely beyond our highest prayers, desires, thoughts, hopes, dreams]."

Despite all of this, I still wasn't at peace. Why? Because my human mind could not understand why *this* (conceiving a baby) wouldn't be what God wanted for me. How this couldn't be in my highest good. How could anything but *that* be the best path for me? My desire to be a mom was through the roof and my ability to be a good one was strong too! What could possibly be *better* than conceiving my baby? It didn't make sense to me.

But remember, God has the bigger picture. He has infinite possibilities that our limited human mind can't fathom.

Even so, I didn't trust God completely to come through for me, so I tried everything I researched and read about because if it was going to happen, by golly, I had to be the one to do it! I took action.

My biggest fear was doubting that God would do what I wanted. How hurtful it must have been to God observing all this, watching and seeing that I didn't really believe He always had my best good in His plans. It probably also upset Him to witness the pain and suffering of His beloved child which He knew could have been diminished with one decision: to rest in my faith, in knowing that God had my back. I could have put an end to my suffering. I could have found my inner peace.

I know that for a very long time I was in that heavy, low energy state because I was determined to fix my problem. That prevented me from accepting my condition completely because, if I believed I could fix it, then it wouldn't be true for me. All of that controlling kept me closed off. There is no peace in controlling; it takes a lot of focus, effort, and energy.

What could be better than having my own baby? I guess I would find out if I surrendered, but I couldn't surrender because I couldn't accept the reality in front of me. The "what is" might be that I will never conceive or birth my own child. Or it may be the reality for right now (this month, this year, but not forever). I resisted accepting this truth because in my mind, *This should not be happening.* It wasn't supposed to be this way. My body should do what it is supposed to do. I should be able to have a baby. I was out to prove it by obsessively focusing on changing this.

Whenever we stamp the word *should* onto areas of our life, we create suffering for ourselves. My husband should, I should, my boss should, my career should, etc. Believing it *should* be different than it actually is steals our joy. When, in fact, whatever *is* happening, is what is supposed to be happening given the sheer fact that it is happening. Many causes and effects came into play for those conditions to arise in a particular way. It wasn't by chance. To be able to accept "what is" is extremely *freeing* and the best place from which to make future decisions because you are not in a resistive state and are more open.

All my energy was going into resisting my truth, with massive effort being put in to making the pregnancy happen. There's

absolutely nothing wrong with taking appropriate action to encourage conception—heck, that's what this book is basically about—but taking action from a place of surrender, and not resistance, is a pretty good way to ensure your manifestation. It's as though you have to be willing to give up what *you* want in order to get it. You need to be willing to really mean those words in the Lord's Prayer, "Thy will be done."

Being able to surrender and let go comes from a high emotional state of openness, allowance, and expansion as opposed to the low emotional state of denial and resistance. When you surrender from this place, you are trusting that you will receive what you are meant to and what is right for you. It may not be exactly what you want in the way that you want, but it will be what you need and is in your highest good. And, if it isn't exactly what you want, you will be okay because something better that you aren't even able to conceive of (no pun intended) is on its way to you as part of God's plan. Being able to trust in this and have that kind of faith is huge. That's a level of certainty, of inner strength through Christ, that no one can take from you and will penetrate any difficult circumstance you encounter. That kind of spiritual health contributes to our healing process because it puts our physical body at peace to rest and recover.

My happiness was tied up in becoming pregnant, so much so that it took precedence in my life. I had to learn to come to a place that my happiness wasn't dependent on *that* happening. I couldn't make this goal of becoming pregnant first place in my life and allowing it to control my happiness and my peace because that's what I was doing. God wanted first place in my life, and my actions and emotional state made it clear that He wasn't. I was so out of balance.

Our umbrella strategy of **I prime the pump, God creates the bump** requires deep trust. You are doing your best (your part, priming the pump) and trusting God to do the rest. Without that trust, you won't have peace because doubt, fear, and worry will still be center stage not allowing your body to truly relax. No one can do the trust part for you. However, you can ask God to help you trust Him and His promises. He will help you. Becoming pregnant is definitely God territory. He is the one who sparks the start of life. So, it doesn't make sense to leave Him out of it. Bring Him into it as much as possible. Talk to Him. Pray to Him. Have a relationship with Him. Listen for His answers on what your next step should be.

Sure, I prayed. I talked and talked, but I didn't sit and listen to God like I'm suggesting to you. It was a one-way conversation most of the time. I wasn't hearing from God because I didn't want to hear anything that might be different from what I *wanted* to hear. I may not have heard from Him, but my dear friend Michelle heard from God very clearly. He said, "Dawn will be a mother, but it won't be in the way that she thinks."

God doesn't cause our problems. He is the solution to them. He may allow certain things to continue in our lives for the benefit of our spiritual growth because he knows how it fits into the bigger picture. Don't misunderstand and think that God is doing this *to* you or punishing you. God is LOVE. Hurting you wouldn't be in His character.

If you are a new believer, God may be waiting for you to partner with Him on your journey. Seek Him more. Ask Him questions. Listen for His guidance. Even if you just call out to Him saying, "God, I don't get this, but I'm going to trust you." And then, show Him that you do. He will be your comfort and strength through this.

If you are a more mature believer and further along in your walk with God, He may be looking/waiting for the spiritual maturity He knows that you have but haven't been demonstrating lately. He may be waiting for you to step up, waiting for you to demonstrate your faith and trust you say that you have by walking the talk via aligned actions that come from surrendering to Him fully. That was definitely me.

If you are a nonbeliever, maybe this is a turning point in your life that God is using for you to come to him and BELIEVE in Him. What do you have to lose? One decision can change your whole life.

Having steadfast faith in a power bigger than yourself isn't a cop-out or taking yourself off the hook. It takes great strength, courage, determination, and confidence. Faith is a potent life strategy. You can't ever lose by putting your trust in God. How about that? Faith gives you so much of what you are looking for on this journey, including hope, strength, certainty, confidence, and peace. All we need to do is be firmly planted in it. Our only certainty in life is what we have within ourselves and our faith in God.

> Patience is not passive; on the contrary, it is active; it is concentrated strength.
> —Edward G. Bulwer-Lytton

Patience

There is no doubt that your patience is being tested during this trying time in your life. According to Merriam-Webster, *patience* is defined as the ability to wait for a long time without becoming annoyed or upset. Patience isn't just about waiting but *waiting well*. You've been waiting, but have you been waiting well?

We receive from God through faith and patience—two extremely challenging traits. Without question, fertility issues demand our growth in both. Perhaps this is where God is asking you to grow, for you to recognize that you can't just rely on yourself for everything; it's time to lean on Him. Time to see that you do need Him in your life. Faith goes hand in hand with patience; if what we wanted always happened right away, we wouldn't need faith.

The strategies throughout this chapter will assist you in being patient. Take part in them. You've got this.

Through the years, people asked me if I'd ever adopt. Adoption felt like I would be giving up on us and on our dream. I couldn't even give that option any attention until I was in acceptance of my reality, which took me a while.

I think I also had the belief that the *ultimate* in motherhood experiences would be to birth my own biological child, and if I didn't become a mother that way, I was missing out on something— that it wasn't going to be as good as it *could* be. Seriously? Societal conditioning reinforces that belief without a doubt.

The belief is faulty and caused me more pain. I wanted to become a mom to love, nurture, and raise a human being who would serve the world in a positive way. Nothing in that statement requires that the human being must be biologically mine or birthed by me.

Once I reached acceptance (which was soon after I had the strong grief release with my friend Kathleen), I was able to come to terms with whether it was more important to physically birth a baby or be a mom. I was ready to take a look at that then.

Reflections and Journal Prompts

What area do you think is the most out of balance for you: body, mind, or spirit?

What do you need to do to **prime the pump** in this area?

On a scale of one to ten (one being not much at all and ten being pretty much nonstop), how often do you think about getting pregnant?

What are those thoughts? Do they have a heavy or light energy to them?

Out of all the strategies in this chapter, which one(s) will be your starting point because you believe it/they will be most impactful for you?

Write a letter to the baby you will mother. Read it daily.

What is your plan to keep your emotional state at its peak regularly?

Create a list of self-care ideas you can incorporate into your day. What brings you joy, even the simplest of things?

Devise a daily routine to incorporate key changes you are making so they become your new patterns. (I.e., before waking, do visualization/read baby letter, breathing/presence, determine who you'll be a blessing to today. In the evening before bed, do gratitude journal, have phone alarm set to assess emotional state, etc.)

Where do you draw your inner strength from? What is your level of faith? How important is it to you and in your life?

Search Bible scriptures or other inspirational literature that address barrenness and fertility challenges to declare and serve as comfort and hope.

SECTION THREE
Guided by the Light

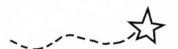

Chapter Eight
Mini Miracles

Live life like everything is a miracle.

—Albert Einstein

What has been invisible to you lately?

In our search to acquire what we so desperately want but don't yet have, we tend to only focus on what we don't have. What we feel cheated out of looms larger. It's as though we put our happiness on hold and don't recognize the joy in what is right in front of us with our search for more.

Is it possible to enjoy your life when you are going through this painstakingly emotional time? Not only is it possible but it's necessary for you to do it in order to bring the abundance into your life that you are seeking.

A surefire way for you to do this is to look for all the mini miracles going on in your life. These mini miracles are moments of grace that reassure you that you are not alone on this journey and that you are surrounded by love. It's God's way of letting you know that He is in your corner and that He hasn't forgotten about you. These mini miracles are God's whispers cheering you on and letting you know that you've got this. It's the encouragement and feeding of your faith that will tide you over until God delivers you from this ordeal.

It is important that you recognize these because it will help to solidify your faith that God is working all of this out for good in your life. He's placing these mini miracle moments along your path to remind you of this.

I had many of these examples of God's goodness during my journey. I'd like to share some of them with you and as you read mine, may they activate you to become aware of the many ways and times God is communicating to you that He is right by your side through this and that you can completely trust Him the rest of the way too.

Mini Miracle #1

I am the middle sister of three daughters in our family. My sister Christie is six and a half years younger than I am. She married her husband a year and a half before I married my second husband, Tom. Incidentally, my first husband disclosed years later in our marriage that he really didn't want children, hence my advanced age in trying to conceive with Tom. Both Christie and I were excited to grow our families with children of our own.

Full disclosure: I wanted to conceive right away given our age (I was thirty-seven and my husband was fifty-two) and given that I had already waited long enough to be a mom because I'd been deceived in my prior marriage. I also hoped I would become pregnant before my younger sister did. Actually, Christie, being sensitive to me and my situation, wanted that for me as well.

Well, that didn't happen. My sister became pregnant two years after getting married, but unfortunately miscarried—a molar pregnancy. About a year later, she was pregnant a second time, again before me. This generated a mix of emotions for me: both happy and excited for her and her husband but also sad and defeated that it wasn't us, still. I knew I would need to intentionally focus on the excitement of Christie's pregnancy and all that it would bring to our lives and not on it as a regular reminder of what I was missing out on and may never experience.

I have to say I was very much looking forward to becoming an aunt for the fourth time (my older sister, Laurie, already had three children), and I was all in to celebrate it with Christie and be supportive. I planned her baby shower and had it at my house. I accompanied her to many of her prenatal appointments. My mini miracle happened during one of her final prenatal appointments. I truly know that this was orchestrated by God.

As the nurse was performing the ultrasound, she asked Christie if she would like to know the sex of the baby. Christie and her husband had always agreed to wait until the birth to find out. Christie answered, "No."

I jokingly said, "But I do."

After the exam, Christie went into the bathroom located inside the exam room to get dressed. The nurse whispered to me to get my attention and motioned to the ultrasound screen that was still on display so she could show me the sex of the baby. We continued to whisper back and forth as I shrugged my shoulders with uncertainty because I wasn't quite sure what I was seeing.

Christie sensed something was happening and shouted out from the bathroom, "What's going on out there?"

"Nothing," I quickly responded, as the nurse and I exchanged smiles.

We left the room with me being none the wiser on the sex of the baby. I did appreciate the nurse's attempt to clue me in despite it being unethical for her to do that. While we were standing at the checkout counter setting up Christie's next appointment, that nurse walked up to me, handed me a sealed white envelope without speaking a word, and then just walked away.

Christie and I both looked at each other immediately realizing what must be in that white envelope. That nurse was certainly taking a risk giving me information the patient didn't want disclosed to someone who wasn't even the patient!

I said to Christie, "I can't believe she just gave this to me. If you want me to throw this away in the garbage right now, I will."

Christie lovingly said, "No. You can be the only one who knows. Just don't ever tell me."

We kept it just between us.

That mini miracle is two-fold. First, the nurse was prompted by God to fearlessly do what she did, and second, Christie selflessly allowed me—alone—to have that special knowledge. This was the starting point of my creating a special bond with my baby nephew. It was such a gift from God that two precious people played a part in. It was something all my own that was just for me to experience. Christie had an intuitive knowing of the value this privileged information would have for me and how it would be such a blessing to me. There was no hesitation on her part to allow me to keep it.

Dante, who is also my godson, is seventeen years old now, and I still have that same white envelope containing the significant ultrasound picture tucked away that I will cherish forever.

Mini Miracle #2

Christie was only permitted to have two people in the delivery room with her when it was time to give birth. Her husband was obviously going to be one of them and she also wanted my mother there as well. My mother is a Reiki practitioner and receiving Reiki while in labor was a bonus for Christie. Words can't describe how much I would have loved to be in the room to witness the birth of my nephew!

When delivery time came around, the nurse ushered everyone out of the room other than the permitted two. My mother went to bat for me and begged the nurse to allow me to be there for the birth as well.

My mother pleaded, "This baby is part her baby too!"

Well, guess what? I was in the delivery room to see my precious nephew be born.

Thank you, Mom. Thank you, nurse. Thank you, God.

Mini Miracles #3 and #4

Halfway into Christie's pregnancy, I resigned from my elementary school counselor position of eight years. The stress of my fertility issues, the numerous failed ART procedures, and my continued ineffective stress management put my anxiety at an all-time high. I was experiencing multiple panic attacks daily at work—all while still trying to stuff my feelings to maintain the level of confidence and competence in my work performance that I and everyone else was used to. I began losing that battle and sought out anxiety medication from my family doctor. The side effects from the medication were challenging, giving me more to overcome each day.

I told Tom how horrible I was feeling, and he suggested that I take a few days off to adjust to the side effects without having the added stress of work. I said, "I'm afraid if I take a few days off, I'll never want to go back."

He comfortingly said, "Then, don't."

My husband's loving support in this matter was truly a gift to me in more ways than one, as you will see. I had wondered for quite some time if the stress of my job in addition to dealing with fertility issues/treatments was contributing to not being able to conceive, and now that work stress would be gone. Plus, I had always planned to be a stay-at-home mom, so at that time, I was all set to go a little early on that end. That was mini miracle number three.

After Christie's maternity leave ended, she needed help caring for Dante once she returned to work. My parents and I both shared in this good fortune. Every Tuesday was my day with Dante. Being in that mommy role with my nephew helped to soften the ache in my heart. The joy, the giggles, kisses, cuddles, the singing and dancing, the playtime, the love, closeness, and connection were just what I needed. It soothed my soul. And it was all possible because I was available to do it since I resigned from my school position. It was most certainly another mini miracle.

Mini Miracle #5

Babysitting for Dante ended up inspiring me to create a product for parents and take it to the marketplace. One day when I was putting two-year-old Dante down for his nap, I began pondering, *Wouldn't it be great to have age-appropriate ideas right at your fingertips to do with your child that were not only fun, but that also promoted their overall development?*

This conception in my mind morphed into a detailed plan and design of yearly wall calendars serving as a combined commemorative keepsake and a parenting resource that provided daily ideas to promote a child's overall development from newborn through five years old. Five separate calendars each with 365 different ideas. Needless to say, I was quite busy not only writing the ideas, but managing all parts of this start-up business of which I had no prior experience. My parenting calendars were mini miracle number five.

These calendars allowed me to use my creativity, my education, my skills, my life experience, but most of all, it beautifully shifted my focus off me and onto something productive designed to help both children and parents. This challenge left little mental energy to feed my constant obsession about conceiving. This was a different "baby" for me to focus on. It gave me purpose and meaning in my life without the stress of work I had before because this was on my terms at my pace.

During that time, I also got the nudge to volunteer for the Make-A-Wish Foundation. I attended training for it and my role was to meet with the parents and their sick children to determine their wish so it could be coordinated. How humbling it was to visit with these families and be an integral part of creating some light in what was such a dark and challenging place for them.

Both the calendar business and the volunteer work successfully kept my focus on others and brought me great joy and satisfaction, which is a desirable emotional state and set point to attract abundance.

Mini Miracle #6

What is extra special about this miracle is that it occurred on my most dreaded day of the year, which may be yours too: Mother's Day.

Attending church on that day was always particularly challenging for me because the priest would generally ask all mothers to stand to receive a special blessing. Trying to conceive unsuccessfully for years and having to stay seated, while so many ladies around me stood up, was excruciatingly painful. I felt like a misfit and not part of the elite group that received obvious recognition for its status. I would fight back the tears, wondering if I would ever get to stand on this special day.

This particular Mother's Day, I was attending mass with my godson Dante and his family at their church, and the priest, as expected, asked all mothers to stand. But he didn't stop there. He asked all godmothers to stand, any woman who was trying to conceive to stand, and any woman who served in a motherly role to a child to stand as well.

With those descriptors, I most certainly met the criteria to be eligible to stand, to be seen, to be recognized, to be celebrated, and to be blessed. Caught by surprise and delight, I stood up proudly as I held Dante's hand. I looked around at so many other mother figures standing. I felt the huge smile on my face and the tears in my eyes again. Only *this* time, the tears were from overwhelming love and not sadness. This had never happened before, and I can't say that I have heard another priest define mother in that way again on Mother's Day. That could only be God.

What I find absolutely fascinating is that in all of the mini miracles I have mentioned so far, Dante played a critical role. Dante, the child I had hoped would be born *after* I had my own child, was exactly what I needed to get me through until *my* time would come. He was the rockstar in the miracles. Christie being pregnant first was the very circumstance God used to help me. What I initially thought was upsetting, God used for so much good in my life. God had the *bigger* picture, and He knew how events should unfold for the highest good of all. This is often what we fail to consider when we are frustrated things aren't happening as we think they should and when they should. There are many intricacies involved that we aren't privy to, which is why trust and faith are so important. Nothing is by chance or coincidence. Life is always working for us even when it seems like it's working against us.

Mini Miracle #7

This miracle encompasses several examples of God making sure I could feel the love and support of close people in my life and be surrounded by it.

Almost no one in my family and friend group could relate to my situation. They all had children or were about to. The statistics indicate that one in eight couples have fertility issues (Cofertility n.d.) but I was like, "Where are they? It's just us as far as I can see." It didn't seem like anyone in my circle was in my position who could truly understand.

God put one in my path. Rosemary was a member of one of my prayer groups and had been down my same road many years before. We had a special connection because she could genuinely relate to my anguish and because she opened my heart to adoption. She adopted her son as an infant and was a living example to me of how beautiful motherhood is through this avenue. Rosemary, along with prayer group members in both prayer groups with whom I worshipped, were integral in keeping my faith strong and lifting me and my husband up in prayer over the years.

Along my six-year journey to motherhood, I held yearly what I refer to as *All-About-You* parties, for five consecutive years. The purpose of this party was to celebrate the ladies in my life who were closest to me, to show them my gratitude, to spoil and pamper them, to do something special that was just for them. Part of the time, we would gather in a circle around glowing candles, seated on our cozy pillows, and share our thoughts on vulnerable topics while each lady was pulled for her turn to indulge in a massage. Being surrounded by that much love and connection was such a support and a reprieve from the heaviness I carried in my heart regularly. I always held the party right around Mother's Day which served as a healthy distraction for me. Once again, my focus shifted to gratitude and to being a blessing to those who have been a blessing to me.

Remember my friend Kathleen who helped me to release my grief? Well, she earned the right for a specific mention in my mini miracles here because that conversation with her was a turning point for me. God spoke through Kathleen by prompting her to say something that enabled me to finally "let loose" with all the grief I had kept stored up. In that moment, as Kathleen held me while I sobbed intensely, I felt validated, seen, and immensely loved. It was then that I was set free.

There are other mini miracles that I could mention, but by now, I think you get the gist. These reassurances, planted at poignant times on your journey, are glimpses of what is to come. Look for the ways that God puts something or someone in your path to comfort you, to encourage you, to distract you, and to feel His presence and His love.

All my mini miracles helped to bring some balance to the emptiness and heartache I was feeling and to show me I could be happy along the way to where I was going.

Mini miracles are the surprises that you may not have directly asked for, but they show up for you anyway. The best things in life just happen without controlling them. For example, someone you meet seemingly by chance at a party gives you a lead on the perfect job opportunity, or the home you have been eyeing for years suddenly goes on sale and your bid is accepted or the serendipitous way you and your spouse found each other.

It's the same way motherhood will happen for you too—that is, if you get out of the way, my dear. God is preparing you to see that with these mini miracles.

Don't miss them.

Look for them.

Notice them.

146

Thank God for them.

It's more of those lighted stepping stones leading you out of the darkness. It's God telling you he sees you, He's got you, and to have no fear. Enjoy and celebrate your life as it is because you can't if you're always looking ahead for what you think needs to be there in order to enjoy it. He's got you covered and is continually working behind the scenes for you. Mini miracles are your proof.

It's only fitting to close this chapter thinking about the original version of the "Footprints in the Sand" prayer by Mary Stevenson. If you have a copy at hand, spend a moment taking it in once again. Jesus can't promise that we won't experience troublesome times, hardship, and sadness, but He does promise us that He is *always* with us, always carrying us.

Reflections and Journal Prompts

What mini miracles of your own have you noticed on your journey?

How many of them can you identify/list?

If you are struggling to come up with any, I'll get you started.

One of your mini miracles is the very fact that you are reading this book. Out of all the books out there on your condition, you are reading *this one*. Why?

How did it come into your presence? Did you just stumble upon it, so to speak?

Did someone recommend it to you or give it to you?

Were you Googling books on the topic and just seemed drawn to this one?

How did it come across your path? It wasn't by accident.

God is whispering to you as you read it and as you do the work on yourself and gain insights.

What does He want you to hear?

To know?

To realize?

To accept?

To release?

To change?

To overcome?

To believe?

To shift?

To surrender?

Keep listening.

Chapter Nine
Support

No road is long with good company.

—Turkish Proverb

This chapter is all about evaluating the quality of your support system and being intentional about how you would like it to look. A positive support system can reduce the effects of emotional stress, amplify your quality of life, and create a buffer against unfavorable life events.

On the flip side, a lack of or a poor level of social support can contribute and lead to loneliness and depression, two emotional states that those struggling with fertility issues can often battle just because of the condition itself. Not having a healthy support system can exacerbate feelings of loneliness and depression. Loneliness increases levels of stress hormones and blood pressure, impairs immunity, and is associated with poor sleep—all things you don't want, particularly when you are putting forth such an effort to bring your body back to complete health and wholeness.

So, let's not downplay the importance of a solid, healthy support system in your life, especially in your current situation. Your support system needs to be one that reduces the stress in your life, not increases it. Unfortunately, many women with fertility challenges feel alone in their struggle and don't feel supported in the way they very much need. Probing questions, unsolicited advice, and strong opinions voiced by family and friends can make you want to withdraw from them completely or minimize contact to avoid additional emotional pain and discomfort in your life. It's a lot to handle when the people you look to for support in your life are causing you more grief. That, coupled with feeling the need to retract from social connections like social media, parties, and events that scream baby-related announcements/reminders or of the inevitable dreaded baby questions asked of you, pushes you further into the depths of feeling alone and not understood.

Some couples decide on the front end to choose not to disclose their diagnosis to anyone at all to maintain their privacy, but this presents challenges of its own with needing to regularly dodge questions like, "So, when are you having children?" or, "When are you going to give me a grandchild? Isn't it time to start trying? You're not getting any younger, you know." So, now you are put in a position of telling white lies to protect yourself from the anticipated emotional distress you thought would have come your way if they knew your truth. That's its own challenge to keep up.

And it's important to note that secrets keep us sick. Not being our authentic selves doesn't feel good because we are out of alignment. You are wearing the mask of "We have no fertility issues; we just aren't ready yet," which couldn't be further from the truth. Living this way is incongruent with what you are seeking. It negates it and it is counterproductive. Not feeling like you can share your reality (for whatever reason) puts you in a shaming/punishing energy that doesn't attract abundance. The desire to keep your truth a secret and consistently perpetuate that secret is completely out of alignment, which is why it feels so lousy. Your intention behind keeping the secret was to avoid experiencing angst that could ensue from others knowing the truth and offering their two cents, but now you have it anyway for a different reason. Keeping up the pretending is emotionally draining and puts added stress on you.

There are ways you can speak your truth and still maintain your peace without having to give up the privacy you desire. We will discuss those communication strategies shortly.

Then, there are some couples (or individual partners of the couple) who are an open book and share what's going on because talking things through is a coping strategy for them. People in their life are aware of the fertility challenges and are privy to a varying degree of these details over time. Some of the informed people may be a positive support while others create more stress with their questions, strong opinions about the couple's decisions, and insensitive comments. This often causes the couple to pull back and limit their sharing and contact, which closes the couple off from a potential circle of support. Isn't it fascinating the strong opinions people have and are inclined to give about something they have absolutely no experience in?

Often, the couple is just left to themselves to cope with the intense array of feelings this condition holds. Sadly, some couples may not even find the support and comfort in each other because the very nature of this problem can drive a wedge between them. If one partner of the couple is diagnosed with a fertility issue, the other may feel a sense of blame or resentment toward that one for the circumstance they are in, and the diagnosed partner may inflict their own self-blame shouldering responsibility for the situation they are in. One partner's desire for parenthood may be dramatically different from the other's and disagreements can arise about what steps they are willing to take to achieve it. Initial agreement to partake in ART can bring its own challenges with the financial strain it incurs, agreeing on the number and type of procedures, and determining when enough is enough if all attempts fail. It's quite a lot to sift through given most couples didn't have these sorts of discussions when they were dating. Rarely is the question asked while dating, "What will we do if we aren't able to conceive?" It's generally not even considered as most are focused on not becoming pregnant until they are ready.

Or you could even be at opposite ends of the spectrum at some point with your spouse with one of you willing to achieve parenthood in a completely different way than the other, like Tom and I were at the three-year point into our journey.

Let's get cracking on creating your positive support system. We'll call this loving group of cohorts your *high vibe tribe* because these people will be the ones that expand your joy, comfort you, listen to you, have your back, and allow you to be yourself without judgment, fixing, or giving unsolicited advice. These are your die-hard supporters that elevate your spirits just by being around them. They are your go-to group and yes, you get to choose them. They aren't automatically in it because they are family or have been friends for years. These are carefully selected people that will positively support you on this journey in all ways.

There is no magic number of members for your high vibe tribe. That's up to you. You may have two people that embody these distinctive traits, or you may have twenty. The important thing is that you know who they are, and you lean on them for this support. There will likely be a time you will be leaned on by one or more of them and you will be able to reciprocate that same support.

Examine all the areas of your life to form your most extraordinary high vibe tribe. Who might they be?

- Family members (which ones?)
- Friends (which ones?)
- Social acquaintances from activities (sports, clubs, fitness center, organizations, etc., that you participate in—anyone fit the bill?)
- Religious community
- Workplace
- Fertility clinic (Perhaps there is someone you clicked with in the waiting room)
- Support groups (online or in person)
- Your spouse/partner (we will cover this one in more detail shortly)
- A fertility coach like myself

My high vibe tribe consisted of my two prayer groups, a few family members, a handful of friends, my boss, and my husband. The type of support and level of support I received within the group varied based on many factors, including frequency of contact, level of closeness, my comfort level, relatability, their role in my life, and my communication style/level of self-expression. It has become very apparent to me that the quality of support I receive from others does not completely rest in their hands. We tend to become frustrated and disappointed when others don't understand us or cut us some slack or if they don't do what we need them to do for us as though they can read our minds. However, we have a responsibility to ask for what we need and to express ourselves in an authentic and respectful way if something hurtful is said or done to us and not stay silent to keep the peace and avoid an uncomfortable situation.

Despite our high vibe tribe's best efforts, there may be times that something is said or not said, done or not done that we may interpret as unsupportive. Your tribe member may not see it that way at all and think they were being supportive.

Keep in mind two very important concepts:

First—Dealing with ongoing fertility challenges and the stress that accompanies them puts you in a heightened emotional state which makes you much more sensitive and vulnerable than you would otherwise be. It's like when we are physically sick, our emotions are right on the surface, and we can be set off easily. We are less tolerant and draw conclusions from that emotional place.

Second—You will need to be aware and understanding of innocent ignorance. Just as you never in a million years thought you would be going through this seemingly no-end-in-sight heart-wrenching situation, and need to navigate this novel experience, it may be all new for your supporters too. They may fumble a bit as they try to figure it out with you. They may never have personally experienced what you're going through, and they want to be there in the best way they can for you, but they are operating from a place of unrelatability so their attempts/assumptions may end up being mistakes. Cut them some slack because they are trying the best they can with the knowledge and resources they have.

If we want to diffuse the level of ignorance and unintended insensitivity out there, we need to stop perpetuating it with our silence, which in turn makes our internal suffering soar. People can't be at fault for what they aren't aware of or don't know. When people know better, they can do better. It's like any unfavorable circumstance; unless someone has been in that situation, they really don't know what it's like. Lack of knowledge begets lack of understanding which begets those flippant comments that streamline their way into every nook and cranny of your heart inflaming the ache.

We can't control what people will say, but we can control how we educate them based on their responses. When someone makes a comment like, "Maybe you're just not meant to have kids," we are typically too hurt to respond, and we shut down and withdraw into our pain. This is understandable but it serves no one. Let's take a new perspective and take solace in knowing that every time you speak your truth—every time you educate someone on your condition or correct someone's misinformation and aren't a victim of their words forfeiting your peace—you empower yourself. You have sparked a ripple effect of shifting the awareness of fertility struggles in support of yourself and your fellow sisters down the road. This is how change happens.

Silence can communicate agreement with what was said. Silence can communicate its accuracy. Silence can infer acceptance of it. Silence can promote more of the same.

So how do you speak up?

Honesty coupled with respect.

For example, if someone says to you, "At least you're having fun trying." This person's intent is most likely to lighten the moment with a spot of humor or to attempt to have you look at the bright side. Let's even assume this person was aiming to be supportive and lift your spirits because otherwise the alternative would be that they are purposely minimizing your situation and invalidating your feelings, which is probably unlikely. I do believe that most people have good intentions to be supportive, helpful, or comforting, but sadly, the reality ends up being the opposite of that.

Why does this happen?

Sometimes people in their discomfort with an emotionally charged topic, and particularly one they are unfamiliar with, speak off the cuff, without any forethought, in an attempt to lighten the mood/conversation.

Sometimes people are genuinely ignorant to the level of distress and despair that struggling with fertility involves and would never realize that their comment would be hurtful. The person in the prior example truly believes that really *is* the good part of not being able to conceive, all the trying. She is completely unaware, having never gone through this.

Sometimes people just like to add their two cents and freely give their opinions and advice. They don't heed the adage "If you don't have anything nice (helpful or useful) to say, don't say anything at all."

Sometimes people's social skills are less than desired, so showing empathy and being a good listener are not in their repertoire.

When we sink into our hurt and shock at these comments, we help perpetuate this ignorance and lack of awareness. If we want change, we need to be the change.

I get it, you're probably thinking, *I have enough on my plate. I'm the one suffering. This person is being a jerk and I need to do something?*

Consider this: How does it serve you well to say nothing?

You conjure up a host of reasons as to what it means that the person said what they did, which are probably inaccurate but nevertheless create distress for you. You increase your stress level with holding on to the emotions that arise within you from the comment, which puts you out of alignment. The person hasn't learned anything and is likely to repeat the action again with you or someone else. And it may be what triggers you to withdraw socially even more, which isn't healthy. That's a whole lot of cons for remaining silent.

The only good thing you get out of staying silent is avoiding the discomfort that you may feel in speaking up against it. Is that worth what you will lose if you don't?

How does it serve you to speak your truth?

Communicating your true feelings in a respectful way is healthy and a form of self-care. It is your right to do this, and it enhances your sense of self-worth. It allows you to process your emotions and not stuff them, keeping you aligned. It is self-empowering and facilitates inner strength and courage which promotes self-confidence. In this way, you are a problem solver instead of a problem maker.

Too often we look to blame others without taking responsibility for our part. Each person has a responsibility to stay in their lane and keep their side of the street clean. If someone shits on your side of the street (with hurtful words, etc.) and you don't clean it up (speak your truth), you are *equally* at fault. It's similar to bullying scenarios where the witnesses who stand by and do nothing to intervene are as guilty as the bully.

Sure, you can choose to disregard this and continue to blame the other person for how horrible they made you feel but, where does that get you except feeling miserable, out of alignment, thinking the world is out to get you, and into a downward spiral?

Or you can take responsibility for your feelings and make a difference through enlightening an uninformed person, making inroads in raising awareness of how infertility really impacts couples, and walk away feeling better than you would have and with affirmation of your self-worth and respect.

I can tell you I have come very far in this area over the years because when I was in the season of my life that you are in now, I truly sucked at it!

What would be an honest and respectful response to that person's comment about it being fun trying to conceive?

I suggest using nonviolent communication (NVC), a technique developed by Marshall Rosenberg. It promotes clear and honest communication with a goal of obtaining harmony.

This is the format that can be applied to structure your response in these situations.

- When I (see, hear, notice) _____ (state what you observe), I feel_____ because I need/value
_____.

- Would you be willing to_____?

Let's put this into action with that person's comment about having fun trying. This is obviously just one of many different example responses of how you could respond using the NVC format.

> "When I hear that comment, I feel really annoyed because there is absolutely nothing fun about scheduled mandatory intercourse that has failed for years on end. I need to feel understood and supported when I share what's going on. Would you be willing to just listen to me vent and not give advice or opinions unless I ask for it?"

This approach is positive, assertive, clear, and doesn't put the person on the defense. Most likely the person will apologize for unintentionally hurting you and you may even go on to have a very productive conversation as a result. You have raised their awareness level, indicated how they can be a support to you/meet your needs, and you can walk away from it at a better place emotionally, knowing you contributed to bolstering their knowledge and empathy skills, enriching your own self-worth.

It's amazing how we tend to judge others unfairly by reading into their comments and behaviors. I could have really used these communication skills with my husband during our fertility struggle.

I vividly remember a comment Tom made to me that really hurt me, and to this day he doesn't know it (he will when he reads this). We were driving in our local area when a call from our fertility clinic came in. We were awaiting results on blood work taken after our IUI to determine whether I was pregnant. The nurse told me that I wasn't pregnant, and I sadly disclosed the news to Tom.

Tom responded, "Well at least you didn't get a call saying you have cancer. Imagine how that would feel."

That comment crushed me because I felt like I wasn't allowed to be sad, disappointed, or angry. Like I had to be grateful I didn't have cancer so I couldn't be upset about what was so important to me in my life. I felt misunderstood, invalidated, and that the news must not be as big of a deal to him, so no wonder he didn't understand how I felt. I felt dismissed, I didn't feel supported, and I didn't say anything. I sank into the hurt of the bad news from the nurse, which was compounded by the hurt of not feeling supported by my husband, although he was none the wiser. Tom came away thinking he was being supportive because I said nothing and that's how patterns begin, and often continue.

When I step outside of this scenario now, given what I know about my husband and men in general, I realize Tom was doing what most men are hardwired to do: fix things, make them better. Tom was coming from a good place. He was attempting to give me a different perspective, a silver lining, because that's a coping strategy he has for himself, so it seemed natural to him to do it with me. Also, unpreferred emotions like sadness are uncomfortable for many people, so it may have also been an attempt to redirect me from it and make it go away for both of us. His words, which I perceived as hurtful, came from a loving place. He is likely to repeat his strategy again because at that time I gave him no indication that it wasn't effective. I read into his comment, and interpreted it as him not caring enough, which in turn, only made me feel worse. I blamed him for making me feel even worse when I was just as responsible for the part I played in it. Let's not fall into that trap.

It's difficult to garner that perspective while in the midst of intense emotion. I invite you to step back and practice empathy as well, by considering all that we have been discussing that can play a role in someone delivering a particular comment. This is a part of processing your emotions, and even if you don't say something right in that moment because it's all too much for you, it doesn't mean you can't say something later that speaks your truth from the heart and serves both of you.

If I had used the NVC model with Tom in that instance, it could have gone something like this:

"When I hear you say something that immediately encourages me to look at the upside, I feel unseen and dismissed. I need you to acknowledge my feelings as valid first. Would you be willing to give me a hug, hold my hand, or cuddle me to comfort me instead?"

So much better, right?

It will take practice to make it become a habit, but the effort will reap many rewards. It may feel uncomfortable before it becomes a habit but push through it because the feeling you get from what you gain will override your initial discomfort big time!

Let's revisit one of the examples from the beginning of the chapter and use the NVC model on how you can communicate to others if you'd like to maintain your privacy and/or minimize discussion about your fertility struggle as a couple and not have to lie about it to do it.

The comment comes in as, "Are you two ever going to make me a grandma?"

Using the NVC model, you could say something like,

"When you ask me questions about having children, I feel aggravated because it's not a topic we want to have open discussion about at this time. I know you are excited about being a grandmother, and I need you to respect our desire to keep this topic tabled for now. When we have something we want to share on that subject, we will. Would you be able to steer clear of questions surrounding it until we feel ready to talk about it?"

I invite you to give this framework a try when situations like these arise and experience what it can do for you and your relationships.

Let's chat about the most important member of your high vibe tribe, your spouse/partner. How would you describe the level of support you give and receive from each other? How would you rate it on a scale of 1-10?

1 = Our fertility issues have driven us further apart. We argue often or withdraw emotionally and seem to be living separate lives. Our conversations and time together revolve around our fertility issues, or we avoid the topic altogether. We don't seem to be on the same page about this.

10 = We have honest, open, supportive lines of communication. We know where each other stands with our plans for attaining parenthood. This experience has brought us closer as a couple. We nurture and prioritize our relationship in the face of our fertility struggle and don't let it consume us.

What score would you give yourselves as a couple? What would need to happen to make it a ten, if it isn't?

Here are some points to consider and be mindful about as you navigate this journey together.

- Men and women are wired differently. There are exceptions, but typically men are fixers and problem solvers while women love to process things verbally to vent, release, and be heard. Men often internalize their feelings which stems from societal/cultural conditioning. They learned to be stoic and that showing emotion is a sign of weakness. It is not weakness, and it is unhealthy to avoid emotions. Men feel they need to be the rock in the relationship. Both partners could be overwhelmed with their emotions, but it presents itself in different ways. One wears their emotions on their sleeve and may be perceived by the other as overdramatic. The other internalizes their emotions and comes off as unaffected by the ordeal or that it doesn't hold the same importance level for them.

Bottom line is our differing patterns for handling our emotions will play out in full force during this challenging time. Being aware of these differences will help you to take things less personally and be more attentive to one another's needs so you are better equipped to support one another.

- Blaming one another will get you nowhere good. Placing fault on the one diagnosed with the fertility issue is unproductive. Don't do it to your partner and don't do it to yourself if the diagnosis was yours. It is not a his or her problem, it's an our problem. See it as that. Make decisions from that perspective.

- Focus on the love you have for each other. You chose each other because of that love, not solely to bear children. Never underestimate the power of healing that can happen on all levels when you love the heck out of each other. Ask yourself when you awake in the morning, What can I do today to make my partner feel happy he chose me to spend his life with? Or What can I do to make my partner's day better today? (And then do it!) You naturally did this when you were dating; bring it back.

- Don't assume your partner knows what you need and how you feel. Take personal responsibility for communicating. Do encourage your partner to share his heart. Create a safe space for him to do that by telling him how much you value knowing how he feels, and how much closer you feel to him when you both speak from your heart. That's intimacy.

- Be mindful to utilize other members of your high vibe tribe for support. Solely relying on your spouse can be a lot for one person to shoulder, particularly when they are dealing with their own emotions as well.

- Pray together.

- According to the scripture Matthew 18:19, "All of heaven waits to release God's best when two agree asking anything in His name, it will be done for them."

- Ask God for what your heart needs. Praying together as a couple is powerful. It promotes connectedness, strengthens your faith, and reduces stress levels. Pursue God with the same tenacity that you do to try to get pregnant and watch what happens. Put much more of your focus on God and His goodness as opposed to your problem.

- Consider enlisting the help of a therapist or fertility coach like myself to help you both navigate this journey.

Reflections and Journal Prompts

Do you feel supported going through this challenging season of your life?

Why or why not?

Who are the members of your high vibe tribe?

How well do you communicate your needs and feelings?

What does support look like for you? (You need to be able to define it so you can ask for it.)

Here are a few examples:

- Maybe you need someone to actively listen to you with no input.

- Maybe you need to hang out with your friends and do something fun without any talk or thought of fertility struggles so your brain gets a break from it.

- Maybe you need your mommy friends to make sure their children aren't the main source of discussion when you're socializing with them.

- Maybe you need one of the members of your tribe to check in on you regularly and directly ask you what they can do to help you.

So, what does support mean for *you*.

Chapter Ten
Happiness

People are as happy as they are committed to being.

—Abe Lincoln

Is there a difference between happiness and joy? These two words are often interchanged. I see them as different. Happiness tends to be something we are in search of—both fleeting and temporary. Joy exists within us, and we can access it whenever we choose, particularly if we become aware of what stands in the way of it.

We often attach our happiness to attaining or having something. Our happiness therefore is situational or conditional. We will even ask, "If I do this for you, will that make you happy?" It's as though there are strings attached to that emotion.

I'll be happy when/if_____ (fill in the blank).

    a.   I get that promotion

b. I move into my larger house

c. I get married (find my soul mate)

d. I have children

Many of us achieve that sought-after circumstance and still aren't happy. We may feel happy for a time, but lasting fulfillment isn't there. Then, we continue the search hoping the next thing will bring that elusive feeling.

a. *You get that promotion, but now you aren't happy anymore because the long hours and rigorous traveling schedule wear you down.*

b. *That larger house takes too much time and effort to keep clean and now you need a house cleaner to help; yes, then you would be happy.*

c. *That husband you thought would make you happy has so many irritating behaviors you wonder why you ever wanted him in the first place. If only he would change, then you would be happy.*

d. *Then there are the couples with children always wishing for the next stage to bring them happiness: when the baby sleeps through the night, when the baby can walk, when the toddler is out of diapers, when the child is out of the sassy teenager stage, when the child drives himself everywhere, when the child finally moves out, if the adult child would just call or visit us once in a while, etc., then they'd be happy.*

We think that feeling we believe exists is contained in a promotion, a mansion, a husband, a baby, but it isn't in those. *It's in us.* We just need to find it again. We have to reveal it to ourselves. When we are able to let go of the need to be perfect, to belong, to be validated, and to perform through achieving, what remains is our joy. Our self-love/self-worth is the pathway to that joy.

Our culture has conditioned us to always want more (like the next shiny object), and we are discontent if we don't get it or until we get it. It has fueled a sense of entitlement. When children do this same thing, "Mom, I want this; I want that" (which really is no surprise that they do this by the way), adults will often say, "You need to be grateful for what you *do* have."

But do we take that advice?

Now, that doesn't mean that it's not okay to want things and to have goals to achieve them, but when our happiness is wrapped up (conditional) in that very thing happening, it is extremely life-limiting and disempowering.

Are you able to find joy in what you have right in front of you here and now, even if you would never receive more?

Because if you can do that (not be dependent on someone else or something else to bring you happiness), you have claimed your personal power and one of the greatest secrets of a fulfilling life. Being able to experience happiness despite your circumstances and not be batted around emotionally by them is how you access joy. That ability to self-regulate in a healthy way (without numbing out) is true freedom.

Joy comes from within. It is our nature and the essence of who we are. We came here with it (which is why it is evident with very young children), that carefree appreciation and love and wonder of life. There is nothing needed to be acquired or participated in by that young child for him to experience joy. Then, that innate joy gets covered up with conditioning and programming from society and those around us. Beliefs and stories are created in our minds, which we view as truth, and we then learn to attach to things outside of ourselves to create the happiness we all desire.

As you release and shift all these layers of cover (which you are doing by taking the action steps suggested in this book), you begin to access this joy that has always been there.

And, interestingly enough, it is this very joy that draws in more abundance to your life. Because remember, outer world is a reflection of inner world, your emotional state.

Some people think they can't be happy or experience joy in the midst of problems or tough circumstances. We think we have to feel bad, as though it wouldn't be right to be happy, during this hard time in our life. Guess what? You have permission to be joyful no matter what is happening in your life. You have a choice. Choose joy.

Being joyful doesn't mean you care any less or that what is problematic has any less significance to you. What it *does* mean is that you are steadfast in recognizing that you can enjoy your life as it is even if it isn't exactly how you would desire it. It means that you have faith. God wants you to enjoy your life, and you can do that when you are able to rest in knowing that He is working on your situation. Enjoying your life as you anticipate the blessing coming in God's way and timing is proof to Him of your trust and that faith gets prayers answered.

> Life is not about waiting for the storm to pass,
> it's learning to dance in the rain.
>
> —Vivian Greene

When you see what is beautiful and lovely in your life now (as it is), you feed that, and more beauty will grow. It's hard to see that beauty when we always want to be somewhere we aren't; for example, when we are stuck in thinking things shouldn't be a certain way. Don't wait to feel joy until your dream comes true. It is the intense power of the joy that you can cultivate now as if your dream has already come true, that will bring to you what is necessary to fulfill it.

When you sustain that feeling of abundance,
you become the condition for all the
abundance that's around us to make itself
visible.

—Dr. Michael Beckwith

"The joy of the Lord is your strength" (Nehemiah 8:10). God's joy is in us as believers. That joy is powerful. If you can keep your joy, it is your biggest strength.

My dear friend, back when I was trying to conceive, I was so guilty of my happiness being dependent on my circumstances and other people. You know I already mentioned to you about my code-pendent tendencies and people-pleasing nature which speaks to that, but you also may recall a clear example of it from the **Story** Chapter when I shared that one of my limiting beliefs was, *I can't be happy if I'm not a mom.* Well, there you have it. I wasn't in control of my joy; it was in the hands of what was or wasn't happening in my life. This belief robbed me of my peace and joy. It's amazing how much our untrue thoughts and beliefs contribute to our suffering and limit the abundance we receive and how disbelieving them can serve us so well.

When you can let go of how things *should be* and move into how *they are*, this is joy. It is being in this state of peace and joy, being grateful in the presence of what is, that will bring you your desires. Find joy in where you are now. If you can't be happy here and now, what makes you think you would be given more? Being able to access this joy is true freedom. When you can find beauty in this place that you don't want to be (in this case your circumstance of having difficulty conceiving), you will find joy. Then you are already living in the joy you imagined you would experience once you conceived, enabling your life to bear witness to that very desire. Because we need to *be* (embody/feel/anticipate) that which we desire to be a match to receive it in our outer world.

It makes sense to do whatever you can to decrease your suffering and access the joy within you. Just decreasing your level of suffering alone moves you towards joy and then there are ways to increase your happiness level. Let's look at some more ways that you can do that.

A lot of what causes our suffering is that we react to our circumstances instead of accepting them. I reacted right from the start of my diagnosis and kept reacting for years. As I denied and resisted the truth that there could be a possibility that I might not conceive a baby, I couldn't relax or be at peace because I had to fight tooth and nail to make sure that I *would* conceive. The thought *It can't be that I can't have a baby* ruled my world. I was determined to prove otherwise. The fight within myself that caused such distress was never going to bring me my baby success. How could it? I was coming from a place of lack and desperation, trying everything I knew to force this baby to be. I was coming from fear with my ego trying to protect me at every turn to keep the identity I was attached to of *needing* to be a mother to feel I was enough and to be fully happy in my life. The tension and contracted energy that ensued from my controlling behaviors to will this baby into being did not allow me to be open to receive it. It pushed my miracle away. Until you accept—truly accept—the truth, you stay locked in that frantic or depressed state or in total despair. That's suffering.

Is there pain in acceptance? Sure, initially, as you grieve what you are accepting, and then it dissipates. But I prolonged my pain through my resistance. Acceptance is the doorway to peace and allows you to relax. Acceptance is recognizing the truth, coming to terms with it, and adapting to it so you can make decisions from a stable place. My refusal (for years) to adapt to this was my nemesis in so many ways.

Could a lack of acceptance be blocking *your* joy?

Emotional and physical pain can cause us to be very self-focused. When we shift our focus to someone else, it lessens our pain and can be very healing as we are intentional about helping them cope with their own pain. Both people benefit, are blessed, and it reduces suffering.

There is a PhD professor of psychology named Sonja Lyubomirsky, who has devoted her career to studying happiness and has written two books on her findings. She suggests that our level of happiness is due to three distinct sources.

50 percent is determined by our genetic set point. Some of us come into the world with a happier temperament than others (just like our physical bodies have a typical weight set point).

10 percent is determined by our circumstances (what our situation is: rich or poor, our physical attractiveness, having a life partner or not, etc.). As we have discussed before, it's not the circumstance itself that is responsible for the happiness or discontent, but rather, what we think about it and make it mean that affects it, in addition to how well we are able to not be dependent on things outside of us to bring us that joy. We chase different circumstances in the hope that we will attain the happiness level we seek which may provide us with some happiness for a short time, but then we become accustomed to it and are on the hunt again. This is why we can see some people in dire circumstances still be positive and upbeat, and on the flip side, some people of significant financial wealth can still feel unfulfilled and be miserable and negative toward life. When you access that joy from within yourself, the circumstance is of little significance to impact that negatively.

40 percent is determined by our actions and attitude and intentionally implementing strategies that raise levels of happiness. Some of which include actions such as reframing the situation, practicing gratitude, performing acts of kindness, engaging in flow activities, and many others. Basically, the strategies you have been reading and learning about in this book would do the trick. Sonja

also found that implementing these strategies, which are in our control, can positively offset a genetic set point/temperament that is wired to be more negative/unhappy. Happy people don't just sit around being naturally content. They take action and have habits in place that sustain that level.

Her findings clearly demonstrate that we have quite a bit of control over the quality of life and level of happiness that we experience. Let that continue to empower and equip you in taking charge of how you experience this journey you are on.

Let me share with you some other strategies I use that make a huge difference. I practice them now in my life and they really work. I didn't do them when I was in your position, but boy do I wish I had. So, I hope you'll take these and run with them.

I remind myself that I have a choice. I always have a choice about what to think about and what to focus on, which in turn affects my emotional state and actions I take from there. That is huge.

If I choose to focus on what I don't have that I wish I did, how things are that I wish weren't that way, all the failures, how I'm getting a raw deal in life, or how unbearable the pain is from it all, I'm going to feel pretty miserable and stressed out. If I *choose* to focus on how I can use this experience to serve me, to learn, to grow, and to become the best version of myself and see what is beautiful that I can appreciate right in front of me here and now, my experience will be completely different. It certainly won't be as sad and frustrating, and my RAS will be looking to match things up in my world to answer these growth-seeking questions being asked. We have so much more power over how our life goes than we realize and that's pretty phenomenal. For this strategy to work its best, it requires you to live consciously, paying attention and being aware of your thoughts so you can shift the "unserving" ones when you recognize them. Don't live on autopilot or you are doomed.

I practice gratitude which we covered in the Strategy Chapter, so I don't need to touch on this too much. Our brain is wired to look for what is wrong so it can help us survive and protect us. Practicing gratitude daily gives that default mode of negativity in our brain less power.

I love this quote by David Steindl-Rast that says, "Joy is the happiness that does not depend on what happens. It is the grateful response to the opportunity that life offers you at this moment." (Intuitive Medicine, June 8, 2020). It is such a beautiful perspective and sums up what we have talked about in this chapter. And that quote comes from a man who spent thirty years on death row for a crime he didn't commit.

I do what I love, and I surround myself with what I love.

- I play tennis.
- I paint.
- I spend time with friends and family.
- I read.
- I snuggle with my dogs.
- I listen to inspiring podcasts.
- I continue learning in areas I want to grow in.
- I watch a few episodes of *Seinfeld*.
- I have fresh flowers in my house.
- I have music I love playing throughout the house.
- I have scents I love permeating the air.
- I do what brings me joy.

Find something that makes you tingle inside and lose total track of time and do more of that. Make sure you are doing a few from your list every day.

I look for the learning opportunity in unpleasant situations. I reframe it and come at it from a different perspective. I try to discern what it is teaching me because we grow the most from painful situations. Might as well find something good from it! That pain can be our greatest gift because we want out of it, so we are more willing to see things in ourselves and our lives that need to change. I know that God will often use these situations for us to learn the lessons that will grow our spiritual maturity for the next level of life we desire.

You may want what you desire yesterday, but God knows the lessons/growth that you need to have in place first. Self-awareness is key to everything. Learn the lesson quickly. Figure it out and then do it. Don't resist. That's wisdom. I love the quote from Wayne Dyer that says, "If you change the way you look at things, the things you look at change" (Brainy Quote n.d.).

I am learning to not want what God doesn't want for me. In other words, I want what His will is for me, otherwise, it may be a disaster or, at the very least, not all that it could be. Just like when you REALLY want to be married and are tired of waiting so you settle for good enough and later realize that good enough wasn't even good at all. Or you really want to purchase that new car, but you know you should really hold off until you are at a better place financially, but you don't want to wait because you really want it, so you buy it. Three months in, you wish you had waited. I am learning to listen to God's promptings and not get out ahead of God because I'm so desperate to have what I want. Trust God's way and His perfect timing. How do you trust? By realizing that the alternative likely won't get you what you are looking for. And by recognizing the many mini miracles that are all around you carrying you, comforting you, and supporting you as you wait, trust, and believe.

I do what my mentor and prominent clinical psychologist Dr. Shefali suggests we must recognize and do. During COVID lockdown, Dr. Shefali would go live with Viral Wisdom videos, and I watched many of them. In one of them she says, "With every get, you have to let." It's the nature of life. We want to control and have things as we want them. But life gives and it takes. There is impermanence. We resist releasing but we still want to get. Honestly, the meaning of that quote is the essence of this book. It's a resounding echo of the title *Free to Conceive*. To get (conceive), you must let go of what is in opposition. You need to clear away what isn't in alignment of what you want in order to make room for what is. If I really think about it, my pain came more from not letting go of/surrendering the dream I had envisioned for myself than receiving the diagnosis itself. As you let go of how you think your life has to go, life appears in the marvelous way it was meant to for you.

True lasting happiness takes residence in both the mind and the heart together. Your mind reminds your heart that your joy exists there and to make the choices that will access it.

> Why be unhappy about something if it can be remedied? And what is the use of being unhappy if it cannot be remedied?
>
> —Shantideva

❧ Reflections and Journal Prompts

How will you access your joy?

What do you need to let go of that is creating a barrier to achieving what you desire? How can you release?

What are you resisting?

What beauty can you identify in your life as it is right now?

Chapter Eleven
Love and Faith

We don't see things as they are, we see them as we are.

—Anais Nin

When you travel this journey from a place of love and surrender, from a place of faith and trust, it can look and feel so differently. That's why the last few years before I became a mother felt lighter to me than the first few years.

Let me show you what I mean.

Shortly after my grief release conversation with Kathleen, something changed in me. I was able to fully accept our fertility challenges and the reality that I might not ever be able to conceive a child.

Did I like it?

Hell no!

But then, I was at least able to entertain that thought being a reality, whereas prior to this point, I avoided it like the plague. I was at a more peaceful place because I wasn't pushing that thought away all the time and resisting it with all my might. I was able to come from a place of self-love and compassion as I considered what our next steps would be.

Once I could fully accept that there was the possibility I would never become pregnant, I was honest with myself, and I knew without any shadow of a doubt that it was way more important to me to be a mother than to conceive a baby. That was a huge realization. I wanted to pursue adoption.

I was ready.

But Tom was not. He still wanted to try on our own without science intervention of any sort. Having a child that was biologically ours was where his heart still was.

Then what?

Well, I couldn't go the adoption route alone. So, there we were, three years into this journey (me now forty and Tom fifty-five), and still no closer to me being a mom.

A few of my friends asked me, "Aren't you going to resent Tom if you aren't ever able to become a mom?"

I said with conviction, "I hope not. I would never want to bring a child into this world that wasn't wanted 100 percent by both parents. Every child deserves that kind of love. We both have to want adoption as our way to become parents. I won't force that to be." (That was already different from how I had behaved the first three years trying to force conception with everything I had in me!)

At that point, I didn't know anything. I didn't know if we would conceive a baby. I didn't know how long we were going to intentionally keep trying. I didn't know if menopause would appear early as doctors had predicted. I didn't know if Tom would ever change his mind and want to adopt. I didn't know if I would ever be a mother. I had to start being comfortable with not knowing. All of it was out of my control.

All of it except my faith. My prayer group had a new prayer now: That God would change Tom's heart toward adoption.

Only God could do that.

Something shifted in me this time around. I believed God would answer that prayer without any doubt or fear. I was free from controlling and forcing and willing things to be my way. I was finally able to surrender. I was finally able to trust that this was in God's hands, and He had my highest good in mind. Oh, the power of surrender. If only I was able to do that sooner! The peace and ease resulting from the freedom of surrender is magical.

My heart had already shifted to wanting to adopt, so it was possible for Tom's to as well. I could relax and go with the flow of life. I didn't bring up the topic of adoption and keep checking in to see if he had changed his mind. I allowed him to be him and me to be me. I respected where he was. I left it alone and didn't try to make it different than it was. No more obsessing and trying to control things. I lived my life positively focused on my calendar business and enjoying my time caring for Dante. Prayers continued and my faith remained strong.

Two more years passed by and still no baby.

One summer day, I walked in the house and saw Tom seated at the dining room table fully engrossed in his laptop computer.

I asked, "What are you doing?"

Tom nonchalantly responded, "I'm just looking up how to adopt a baby from Columbia." Like it was no big deal, like it was something he did all the time.

Well, maybe he did, and I just didn't know it, but it seemed totally out of the blue to me!

I was stunned and could barely get out the word "What?!"

We continued with our conversation after I pinched myself to make sure I wasn't dreaming. I asked Tom with extreme curiosity, "What changed your mind?"

Tom replied affectionately, "Seeing how you are with Dante all the time. You have so much love to give. You *have* to be a mother."

Sweeter words could not have been said. It was as if he was saying it's been enough time now putting off the inevitable, our destiny.

Once again, Dante was the rockstar of another mini miracle. What is that, like six miracles for him now? He really packs a punch! God got a lot of bang for his buck having Christie become a mom first! God used my endearing relationship with Dante, the child who came first, to be the very reason to shift my husband's heart toward adoption and make me a mother. Never doubt God's ways. He knows exactly what He is doing.

Then, with me at forty-two years old and my husband at fifty-seven years old, we were ready to embark into the unchartered territory of adoption.

My experience with adoption was completely different from my experience of trying to conceive because I was different. They are both avenues to become a mother permeated with so much that's out of control, but one felt much better for me because I utilized many of the tools contained in this book without even knowing it at that time.

Let's face it. Adoption is riddled with many fears of its own, like:

- Where do we even begin with this comprehensive process?
- Will we be approved?
- Will we ever be matched with a child?

- How long will we have to wait?

- Can we afford this?

- How do we navigate all the shady stuff that goes on with baby buying?

- What if we get so close and the birth mother changes her mind and keeps the baby?

All those fears and unknowns were there with adoption, just like trying to conceive has its own set, but this time, I felt peaceful.

How was I different? I was peaceful.

Why was I peaceful? My faith was strong. Way stronger than before. It allowed me to surrender and not obsess and control. I may have wavered in my faith to conceive a baby, but I never wavered in my faith to become a mother. I had a knowing deep within me, a certainty that couldn't be shook, that *this* was my path to motherhood. That *this* was God's plan for me.

I met with challenges right from the get-go when two out of three adoption agencies I contacted burst my bubble on the likelihood of us getting matched with a newborn because of our age. Both these agencies stated that there would be a very low probability of birth mothers choosing us because they would view us as grandparents to their child and would prefer younger adoptive parents. Given the age of the birth parents, they themselves could have been considered our children and the birth mothers don't like that perspective.

When fear and discouragement started to creep in after these calls, I didn't let it take over. Thoughts like, *Maybe we are too old to start this process* or *Maybe parenthood just isn't meant to be for us* and *Now my age is going to prevent me from adopting too?* or *It shouldn't be this hard to become a mom.* These thoughts came in, but I didn't give them any life because this time my faith overpowered my fear and doubt. I didn't attach to how this was all going to work out, I just knew that it would. That belief was stronger than any other. My faith kept me taking the next step forward and trusting. Because I was in my heart space, peaceful and aligned, I could trust the next step to take.

I called the third agency I was referred to and addressed the age issue head on at the beginning of the call. Barbara Casey, the adoption lawyer and owner of the agency, assured me that our age wouldn't be an issue at all for creating matches. She said that in fact many birth mothers actually prefer an older couple who is more established in their relationship together and has more financial security. This was music to my ears and the music got even sweeter when she said that the average amount of time it took for couples to be matched with their baby was nine months to a year.

Here's how incredibly amazing God is: Nine months from the day we signed on with this agency, nine months, the length of a typical pregnancy, Tom and I held our newborn baby girl in our arms. A baby girl that we witnessed be born. A baby girl that my husband was able to cut the umbilical cord for. A baby girl that we *had* to name Faith.

We weren't just matched in that quoted time frame; we were parents beginning our lives as a family of three all within nine months. God moved quickly this time around because I didn't interfere. I surrendered. I believed. I trusted. I did my part and I let God do the rest. I had faith. I acted "as if" and my thoughts, words, feelings, and actions were aligned with my faith. My faith brought me Faith on September 13, 2010. Faith is the ability to manifest evidence of it in your life.

I really did act "as if" and made some bold decisions based on my belief that I was going to become a mother without a doubt. I ordered all the baby room furniture. I had a muralist come in and paint a full-sized giraffe on one wall of the nursery and a large tree on another on which we hung wood shelves to give the look of dimensional branches.

I had such fun scouting out decor ideas to make this a magical room for my baby who I knew was on the way to me. That's right, fun! My emotional state was one of joy, anticipation, and love which was a match to what I most desired, a baby. As you know, that's not the emotional state I typically had while trying to conceive for years. I was often on edge, desperate, controlling, and fearful.

God loves to create synchronicities. On March 23, 2010, our baby furniture was delivered. We weren't yet matched with a baby, but the room was ready for one! Later that same day, arrangements were made for us to speak with a birth mother who had chosen us as potential adoptive parents. If both parties felt good after the call, we would then be considered an official match and be able to proceed with the adoption process. So, on March 23, the day baby furniture was delivered, we were matched with our baby who was due to be born in six months.

We even celebrated with a baby shower in July. Was it a risk? What if the birth mother changed her mind and we would have to drive all the way back home to Pennsylvania from Texas empty handed surrounded by baby paraphernalia everywhere we looked? This thought entered my mind when contemplating doing the shower before or after the baby was here and my faith won. My faith made the decision with no wavering. My faith won every time, the whole time. God rewards that kind of faith. Everything fell into place. It was God driven. I just followed His lead.

I often wondered as we were going through the adoption process if I would still yearn for a biological child of my own. Would that ache really ever go away? When we are in God's will, His grace is upon it. He took care of that. That ache was completely gone from the moment I held Faith in my arms. She was mine; there was nothing missing except that soul-searing ache that thankfully never returned.

I have heard that love is the answer to every problem. Every problem. That love always has the last say and it's a sure thing.

Love never fails. The energy of love is so powerful and healing that tremendous shifts can occur. We tend to think of it as only an emotion, but in order to harness its full power it needs to be a way of life: how we lead our life, with love and not fear.

Unfortunately, fertility challenges can bring about a lot of fear if we live unconsciously. It has so much involved with it that doesn't feel loving at all.

We detest our bodies for not performing reproductively how they were designed to.

We wonder if we did something to deserve this curse.

We think we are abnormal and defective and question our worth.

We feel misunderstood, lonely, unseen, shamed, and excluded.

We feel pressured by our biological clock or by our family, and in turn, can put pressure on our husbands to perform like a machine as opposed to our lover.

I invite you to operate from a place of love throughout this fertility journey: love for yourself, love for others, love for the gifts that this struggle to conceive a baby will award you.

The English Proverb "You catch more flies with honey than with vinegar" stands true. We will experience more success in life being loving (sweet like honey) than being hurtful, unkind, or harsh (vinegar).

How can you bring some *honey* into this journey? Let's transform this fear into love because that is the answer. Holding the question in your mind, *What would love look like right now?* will help you do that.

Instead of detesting and hating your body for letting you down, what would showing it love look like?

How about sending love to all your body parts, organs, systems, bones, muscles, cells, etc., that are functioning well and continue to support you in so many ways on a daily basis that we tend to just expect and take for granted? Send love to the system/s (reproductive, endocrine) that are imbalanced so they can heal. Love your body *even with* this condition because it's telling you something. Have compassion for yourself. How about being grateful for the message this fertility struggle (imbalance in your body) is sending you so it can be the catalyst for your awakening and emerging. Thank your body for alerting you to what needs to change mentally, physically, spiritually, and emotionally so it can function optimally for you in all ways and that you are doing your part to respond with love to that message alert.

How would healing that be to your body? Instead of fearing this condition and focusing on how you can fix it/get rid of it/deny it, ask what your body needs from you. Ask what your body needs to heal and trust your intuitive knowing. What will bring it to a place of harmony? Do what will nurture and nourish you, heal you, and help you. Forgive yourself for being angry at your body. Whatever you do to support your body, do it from a place of love, not desperation, resistance, or anger. Show your body honor, care, and love. That is what it is needing most right now because it is hurting. The healing energy of love will be transformative for it.

What if, instead of berating yourself for what you must have done to deserve this curse, you look at the situation through the lens of love? You realize that God (life) isn't doing this to you. God loves you and He has your back. Perhaps, because He loves you, He is using this season of your life to bring to your awareness what needs to shift/change/be recognized in your life that may have set this condition in motion and has kept it there. Decide to look at how this condition/circumstance in your life could be working for you as opposed to being done to you. It's a curse looking through the lens of fear. It's a gift looking through the lens of love. Fear keeps us stagnant. Love moves us forward.

What if instead of seeing yourself as unworthy, abnormal, and defective you see yourself as God sees you? God is love and you were made in His image. The master of the universe created you and wants you here. Your worth is a direct result of that alone. You came from Him, so how can you be unworthy? It is this connection to God that is your true worth. But you have to believe in that worth and claim it. You have to recognize that. No one can do that for you. This may be the root for your growth that needs to occur to confidently support the dream you are seeking to be fulfilled.

What if instead of being envious and jealous of all the mamas around you having baby showers, posting baby announcements, and celebrating their little one's birthdays, you came from a loving place instead? The fact that there are all these babies means that they are in abundance for you to have. There is no lack. Celebrate all those babies as they are God's beautiful blessings that were given by grace and weren't earned; that's love. I know it hurts inside when you want so badly what everyone around you seems to have, but the vinegar (jealousy, anger, envy, holding yourself back from celebrating their joy) keeps you in resistance and not open to receiving this abundance. You can be sad or disappointed for yourself and still be happy for them.

Being a mother begins in your heart. You have so much love in your heart with your desire to mother a child. You are already on your way. Use that love to anchor you and it will continue to expand. That pure intention of love you have for them will have a positive effect on your nervous system. The energy of celebration, joy, and love is one you want matched in your outer world. Don't hold it back. Share that supportive motherly love with those around you having babies. Show your love for their little miracles. Show your love for the mamas who were gifted these miracles. Your time will come. And love is the answer.

Instead of demanding your spouse/partner abide strictly to your ovulation schedule so no chances are missed for baby making, let love and enjoying each other be your guide for baby making and then it won't feel like a chore. Fear is what makes us obsess over our cycle and be devastated if our spouse wants to skip a "prime" day. Having to control everything is fear based. Ironically, that control we put in place that we think will get us closer to what we want is the very thing keeping us from it. Have fun, be romantic, sexy, and creative, just as you were before you two were trying. Rekindle that. Any decision we make from fear is the wrong one. And it feels so heavy, which is a clear indication of it being fear. Ask yourself, *What would love look like in this situation? Am I making this decision out of love or fear?* Love feels light—love feels right. Choose love.

The space I was in from the point at which I chose adoption was a space of love. I lovingly waited and let Tom find his way on his own and in his own time to meet me there. My decisions made during the adoption process were ones made from love and not fear. That's why the process felt so good and was in flow.

When you make your decisions along this motherhood journey and in life, make them from your heart space, from an emotional state of love and peace, so you are intuitively guided and in your higher self as opposed to your lower self in fear, worry, or desperation. In this place, prayerfully ask God what He wants you to do and the peace He provides you with will be your guide. The same goes for your intentions. What you want and desire in your life needs to have the energy of love infused in it, not fear. Make sure the prayers you offer to God don't just contain the what but also the why. The why denotes how it will glorify God, and the why holds the intentional energy of love. The what and the why that isn't selfish (from the ego) or only inward based get answered. God always approves of an intention with the basis of pure love.

Recognize the love that is all around you all the time. Unconditionally. Proof of God's love for you is evident in the sun, the flowers, the beauty of nature, the power that is breathing you. That breath is life. You are being loved in every moment because God chose you and wants you here for a specific purpose.

I love Rumi's quote: "And still, after all this time, the sun has never said to the earth, 'You owe me.' Look what happens with love like that. It lights up the sky." (Pass It On n.d.)

Just as you can rely and trust that the sun will rise every day and that you will breathe by way of this power greater than you, you can also trust that this God is supporting every aspect of your life in this same way whether they are visible to us or not. That is His love for you.

The more we are grateful and see the love in front of us now in this present time and everywhere, the more we will be given things to love. How are you treating the people God has already placed in your life to love? How are you showing your love for God?

There is a saying that goes: Love brings up everything unlike itself to be healed. This is an invitation for you to be kind, loving, and compassionate with yourself in all ways. The more you take care of yourself body, mind, and spirit, the gentler you are with yourself, the more honest you are with yourself, and the more forgiving you are toward yourself, it may stir up all the other emotions lying dormant that need to be released. Heal what you may not even have realized you have been holding on to.

Have you ever noticed when someone is angry/frustrated and their words toward you come out venomous or harsh, because they are hurting? And when we are hurting, we are most in need of receiving love. If you react to the person in that same manner because you feel offended, war ensues. If you respond to them with love by offering a hug, meeting them where they are, and connecting with how they are feeling and not taking it personally, it creates a safe space for the love to be accepted and healing to happen. Do this for yourself and feel the difference.

I find the work of Dr. Kelly Turner fascinating. She conducted research in ten different countries over a period of ten years that analyzed over 1,500 cases of radical remission of cancer. Her book summarizes this research. She identifies nine essential factors of spontaneous remission with cancer. This refers to someone who heals from cancer in a statistically unlikely way without the aid of conventional medicine or when conventional medicine has been unsuccessful.

Out of the nine essential factors, only two of them were physical. The first was that patients radically changed their diets (such as reducing wheat, sweets, meat, and dairy, increasing fruits/ vegetables, drinking filtered water, and eating organically). They basically eliminated things that would increase inflammation in the body. The second was taking herbs and supplements unique to their needs.

The other seven factors were mental, emotional, and spiritual which, as we know, are closely tied to the physical body. Here are the other seven:

- Increase positive emotions
- Release suppressed emotions
- Follow intuition
- Deepen spiritual connection
- Love from friends and family
- Finding strong reasons for living
- Taking control of their health (shifting from feeling helpless and taking back their power) (Integrative Cancer Review n.d.)

I'm sure these same factors would hold true for healing many diseases. Fertility challenges encompass all areas: emotional, physical, mental, and spiritual. It only makes sense to heal it from a wholeness approach.

Reflections and Journal Prompts

What does your mind, your body, and your spirit need to create the best environment for a baby to come and flourish?

Are you making decisions along your journey based out of love or fear?

What would this fertility struggle in your life look like if you were to operate from love and not fear? How would you think about it? How would you feel about it? What would be different in your actions and decisions you make toward yourself, others, and your fertility treatment approach?

If you would see yourself as God sees you, what would you do differently? What steps would you take from that place?

Chapter Twelve
Freedom

My mother would take the Band-Aid off, clean the wound and say, "Things that are covered don't heal well." Mother was right. Things that are covered do not heal well.

—T. D. Jakes

You are on a journey to motherhood and this book has also taken you on a journey of its own, a journey of self-reflection, self-understanding, self-growth, and transformation. This is an ongoing journey.

I am still on it. It's the path I choose so I can continue to live my best life.

The greatest gift you can give yourself and others in your life is the highest version of yourself. Your doing that will be the greatest gift you can ever give to your baby.

My hope is that, as a result of reading this book and doing the work contained in it, you will break the stronghold that your fertility challenges have over you. That's freedom.

To be free means to not be determined by anything. You don't let it control or define you. It means you are released from the confinement of this condition. It means that you are relieved from something burdensome and unpleasant. That nasty (i-word that I won't say) diagnosis and prognosis doesn't define who you are or what your future as a mother will be. You aren't a victim who succumbs to that label. The prognosis is up to you and from that stance you take your power back. You get to decide what it means that it hasn't happened yet. You get to choose who you want to be on this journey and how you want to feel. You get to define how motherhood will look for you. You have the tools now to direct and create your life as you conceive it to be. You get to conceive something new based on the new you to rise to the next level of your life. Consciously chosen conception is very empowering.

You get to choose what you will think, how you will feel, what your attitude will be, how you will act, and how you will show up during this season of your life. You get to conceive and choose the experience you want to have.

Will you see this problem/situation in your life as one of despair and punishment? One in which you are helpless and there is just darkness? Or will you choose to see it as an opportunity to grow through what's been brought to your awareness and learn the lessons to prepare you for the blessing you desire? Will you choose frustration or joy? You are free to choose. What you choose will bring outcomes that match accordingly and create your reality.

Imagine that you are carrying a backpack on your back. You have been carrying this backpack around for years and, with struggling to conceive, it seems to have only gotten heavier. When you first started reading this book and before you started doing the work involved, the backpack was extremely heavy and weighed you down. It was filled with heavy rocks. These rocks symbolize what has been standing in the way of you achieving what you most desire, a baby.

Throughout the chapters in this book, you have been doing personal excavation work like digging deep to uncover and expose what hasn't been serving you well and what has been keeping your body out of balance and you misaligned. As you uncover, shed, and release this, and in tandem, cultivate that which will serve you, you allow true beauty to emerge. The highest version of you. What's been revealed and exposed brings you back to harmony, balance, and wholeness. What's left is pure—authentic—and can blossom and grow and expand. It is freedom.

This transformation can only happen with awareness, by being fully transparent and honest with yourself. As they say, the truth shall set you free. Keeping the blinders on only keeps you stuck. Change can only happen from this place, and it takes courage to overcome your fear, to be open, and to see things differently. You can't be free from anything until you recognize it and have that awareness. It takes courage because you are leaving what's familiar and going into the unknown with new habits, thoughts, beliefs, and actions. But you trust that going forward into the unknown as the transformed you trumps the certainty of what is familiar and comfortable in where you are now. Becoming a better version of you, although it may feel strange at first, beats the comfortable status quo. Nothing changes if nothing changes.

Carrying that heavy backpack around everywhere you go is constricting and limiting. That backpack is weighing you down and closing off your womb. Picking up this book to read and doing the work signaled that you have had enough of this burden, and it was time to free yourself. You can't truly be free to conceive until you recognize what is creating a barrier to it. Once you know and acknowledge it, you overcome it to experience that freedom. You end up getting out of your own way.

Let's take the rocks out of your backpack, one by one, so you can see what you have released, let go of, transformed, and *freed* yourself of.

Imagine that each rock you pull out signifies a barrier that no longer exists in the way it once did. Good riddance to:

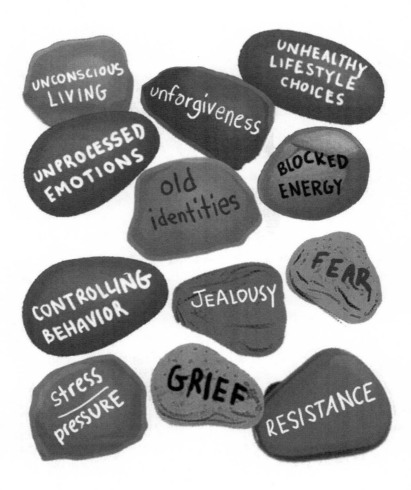

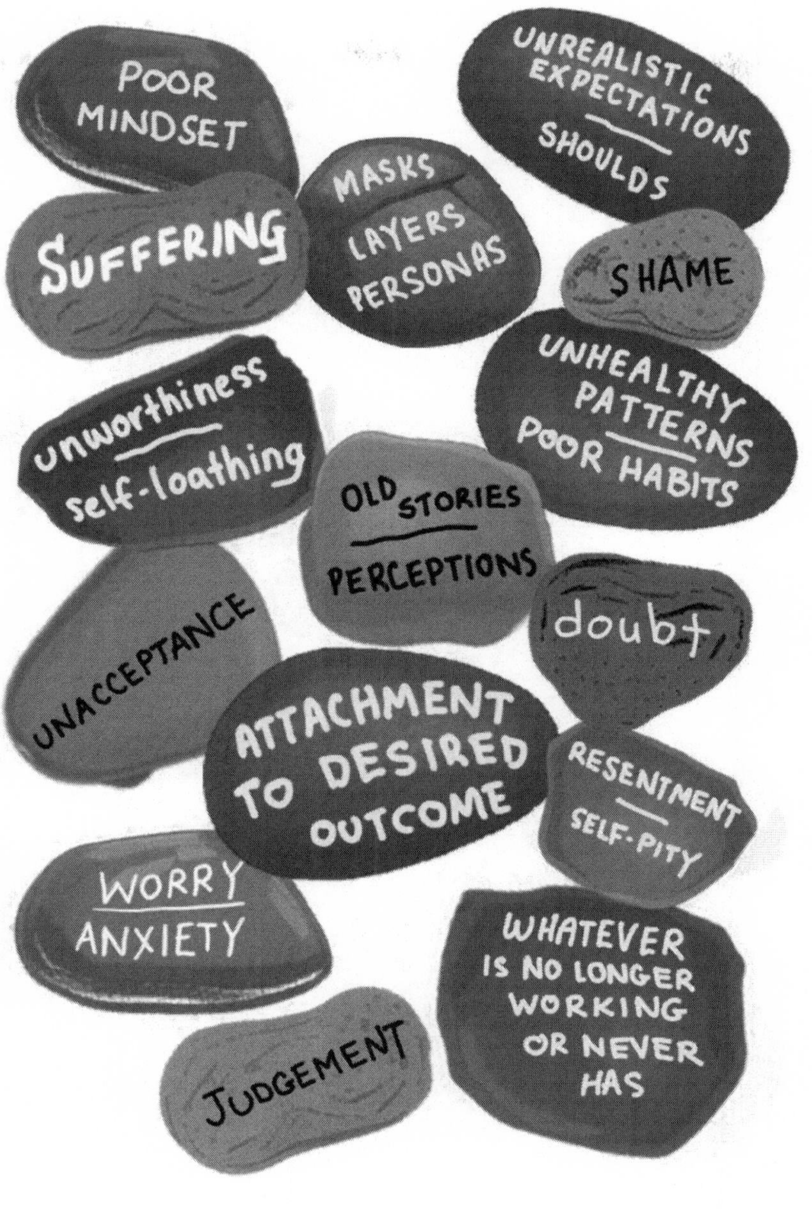
POOR MINDSET
UNREALISTIC EXPECTATIONS
SHOULDS
MASKS
LAYERS
PERSONAS
SUFFERING
SHAME
UNHEALTHY PATTERNS
POOR HABITS
unworthiness
self-loathing
OLD STORIES
PERCEPTIONS
doubt
UNACCEPTANCE
ATTACHMENT TO DESIRED OUTCOME
RESENTMENT
SELF-PITY
WORRY
ANXIETY
WHATEVER IS NO LONGER WORKING OR NEVER HAS
JUDGEMENT

Wow! No wonder you felt so weighed down! As you released these rocks, you cleared the way of what was not in alignment for you, for what is. You have freed up space to be open and ready to conceive. Your backpack is super light now. It is open and expansive. It is open to receive. The person carrying it is free. Free to receive. Free to conceive.

Not only did you experience this freedom by releasing and letting go of the struggle and what doesn't serve you in your life or in attaining what you desire, but you also experienced it by cultivating more love, peace, joy, trust, faith, and gratitude in your life. These, combined with claiming your self-worth and your authenticity, are the truest sense of freedom.

Basically, throughout this book, we have been working on closing the gap between where you are and where you want to be. The Five-Point SuperStar System and subsequent chapters in this book have been your guide to do that. Hopefully, you have discovered what your missing pieces are. Your freedom lies in addressing the root cause of your condition. What area do you need to address the most even though all five points of the star really play off one another?

I struggled to surrender because of my fear of conception not happening if I didn't try to control the situation. The intense fear stole my faith. The fear stemmed from my limiting beliefs (my story) and how my worth was wrapped up in the identity of being a mother and a high achiever. My limiting beliefs were rooted in my poor level of self-worth/self-love. Working on the *Self* part of the SuperStar System would have been my starting point if I had this book back then and in doing so it would have had ripple effects to help shift my story, my state, and my being able to surrender. Owning your worthiness is really the key to everything you want because it puts you in the state to draw it in to you. Claiming your worth is where your joy is. It allows you to be truly authentic and experience freedom like no other.

This book pretty much leaves no stone unturned when it comes to what could be the missing piece in your fertility puzzle. Instead of working so hard on becoming pregnant, you have been encouraged and led to put that energy into working that hard on yourself. It brings rewards of all sorts. It's common to just look at the physical barriers getting in the way with fertility and addressing those. We tend to overlook the most critical piece of the puzzle, ourselves, and how we sabotage manifesting our desires by getting in our way. I am so proud of you for lifting the veil, getting real, and participating intentionally in the life you want. You did this with utilizing the Five-Point SuperStar System.

I am so proud of how far you have come since we started this journey together. You were far from free then. You were full of fear and felt a lack of control over your situation. You were constrained by the powerlessness you felt from your diagnosis. You were heartbroken, grief-stricken, angry, and frustrated. You felt inadequate, alone, misunderstood, uncertain, defeated, resentful, and jealous. You may have been unable to surrender and forgive. Your body was sitting with suppressed feelings from the past and present. The way you felt about yourself was very different. The stress from limiting beliefs you held as well as old stories, perceptions, patterns, habits, and mindsets was keeping your body out of balance.

Now, you are free to be the true you, to be authentic. You are free to accept and surrender. You are free to believe, to trust, and to be honest with yourself. You are free to feel fully and express yourself. You are free to tell a new story, to experience peace, to be happy, and to live your life fully. You are free to conceive in all ways.

Do you win if you can't lose? I'd say so. A winner, that is you on this journey. With or without a baby, you have succeeded. You have succeeded because of who you have become as a result of the work you have done along the way. You take this transformation with you wherever you go. And it may just be what allows you to be free to conceive your baby. You are showing God you are ready.

I want to leave you with a metaphor that can serve as a reminder for how to be on this journey to motherhood and on your whole life journey as well.

See the image of this palm tree. The palm tree represents you.

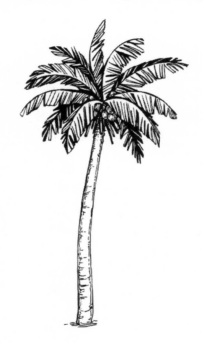

The **roots** of the palm tree signify that you are rooted and grounded in self-love, which means you are rooted in God's love. You know who you are, a facet of the divine whose worth does not need to be earned, proven, or measured by anything or anyone. That self-love allows you to receive God's love for you and you do life together with Him from this perspective. This gives you trust, faith, and certainty that all of life is unfolding *for* you and not *to* you. Make God your priority. Think more about Him than your problems because He is the solution. This is your strength to withstand the storms of life and thrive.

The **trunk** of the tree symbolizes living consciously, attentive to and aware of your thoughts, beliefs, mindset, attitude, and emotional state so that you are in charge and creating the life that you want. It's you, executing the knowledge and tools you have learned.

The **leaves** (palm fronds) represent being in flow with life. You sway in the breeze with no resistance to what is happening in your life. You practice presence. You release the struggle in trying to control situations and surrender to what is, so you can remain in an open and expanded state. These leaves symbolize your freedom.

Living in the moment and not in the past or worrying about the future is all we really have. This moment is what is real. The future is a thought, and the past is a thought we conjure up in our mind. It doesn't mean the past didn't happen—it did—but it's not happening now until you choose to experience it from thoughts you think in the present time. Same thing applies with the future: the what if's that you fear are not real. Some of them may actually happen down the road, but if they do, it will be in present time. It's not now. What's happening right now is truth and real and allows us to be free from emotional pain. When you don't like how you are feeling, assess what your thoughts are and in what time (past, present, future). Bring yourself back to presence with focusing on your breath.

The **fruit** that grows on your tree represents the good fruit that you will bear in life. It's you, shining your light on others in the world as a reflection of who you are inside. Your fruit consists of your personal growth, your character, your service to others, your attitude, sharing your unique gifts and talents you have been blessed with, your authenticity, and all that comes from your heart. This fruit may also symbolize the fruit of your womb that you conceive. You will bear good fruit staying intentionally connected to God.

The **shedding of dead palm fronds** signifies you releasing that which doesn't serve you, just as you did with the rocks in the backpack. It's the continual cycle of pruning to remove what isn't desirable so it can stimulate more growth in order for you to enjoy your most abundant life.

Be the tree.

Hold the image of this palm tree in your mind and embody it. Let it be a reminder of the quality of life you can choose to have as you do your part in partnership with God.

This moment is bittersweet for me because it's time for me to bid you a fond farewell. I will miss our time together, but I am beyond excited to see what is coming your way. I'll say so long, as my late grandmother always would, by offering up a special prayer for you.

Dear God,

Thank you for your precious daughter reading this prayer right now. You know her heart. You know her deep pain and her struggle. Thank you for her willingness and courage to look within herself and dig deep to discover her answers to the questions she has as to why she hasn't conceived a baby yet. Keep encouraging her to seek you and to continually strengthen her relationship with you.

Let her feel your comfort. Fill her with your amazing peace. I pray that she receives your love fully because she knows she is part of you and worthy of that love as your chosen special daughter. Assure her that since you placed this strong desire to be a mother in her heart that you will guide her to the fulfillment of it according to her highest good. Remind her that your will is what will ultimately satisfy her.

Surround her with encouragement and love and fill her with your wisdom. May this precious woman feel your joy each day as she patiently waits for your deliverance.

I pray this in Jesus's name.

Amen.

Dear Soul Sister,

It has been my absolute pleasure, privilege, and honor to walk arm in arm with you on this part of your journey. May you be blessed in ways you couldn't even conceive in your wildest dreams.

All my love,

Dawn

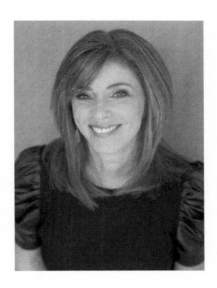

About the Author

Dawn Williams knows the pains, sorrows, and challenges of the conception journey first-hand. Based upon her own experiences, the women's wellness coach developed a transformative approach that is specifically designed to empower those who struggle with fertility issues. Dawn is praised for providing a loving and comforting approach that mixes the practical with the spiritual. She supports women in taking charge of their fertility and restoring their sense of inner peace as they journey towards making their dreams come true.

Dawn has a master's degree in counselling psychology and is a certified love and authenticity practitioner. Her unique perspective and approach to overcoming fertility challenges considers more than just the physical reasons that impede conception and focuses on aligning mind, body, and spirit to bring the body back into alignment so that it can do what it is designed to do. Her compassionate approach supports her clients in transforming their relationship to fertility challenges enabling them to let go of the struggle and gain a sense of lightness and joy. Dawn resides with her beloved husband, daughter, and three dogs in Eastern Pennsylvania.

Extra Support

Sometimes you need more. Maybe you have made some inroads but need the help of someone who has traveled your road to help you go deeper and close the gap even more. I can honestly say the depth of personal growth I have acquired and shared with you here has been due to the help of incredible mentors and their ongoing support. I didn't do it alone. You may also need the support of someone who can lead you where you are unable to go by yourself so you can truly make the leap from just consuming all this information to implementing it to create change. If that is you, know that I am here to coach you further in a way that can best meet your needs. I offer a complimentary 1:1 Discovery Call to determine if we are a mutual fit to work together and what would be your best next step based on programs that I offer. Go to the link below to book your free call.

YourFertilityAngel.com

Nothing would give me more joy than to hear from you as to how this book has impacted you. Maybe you will share how you have personally grown in so many areas, maybe you will send me a picture of you pregnant, maybe you will share how much better you feel as you wait on God's timing, maybe you will share that you are adopting, and maybe even you will send me a picture of you with your baby. Oh, how that would touch my heart in ways you can't even imagine.

For more great books from Gracelight Press
Visit Books.GracePointPublishing.com

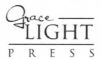

If you enjoyed reading *Free to Conceive,* and purchased it through an online retailer,
please return to the site and write a review to help others find the book.

Made in the USA
Middletown, DE
27 July 2023